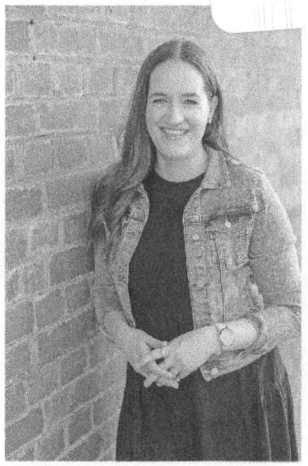

Lauren Novak is an award-winning news and features journalist of more than two decades. She lives in South Australia with her partner and their two children.

For updates on Lauren's writing, visit laurennovak.com.au or follow her on Instagram, @laurennovakwrites.

PRAISE FOR *MELTDOWN*

'This generous book is like a soothing balm for any mother who is feeling overcome by rage. If only I had it to guide me at the beginning of my parenting journey. I'm buying it for every new mum I know'
Penny Moodie, author of *The Joy Thief*

'Motherhood in the 21st century is much more demanding and challenging for so many reasons and *Meltdown* written by Lauren Novak is a deep, honest and raw exploration of the emotional costs, especially mum rage. With her own story as a foundation, she weaves the research, the science, the psychology of stress and female hormones, with poignant true stories from mothers everywhere to make sense of the hot, unpredictable meltdowns. Every mother needs to read this book because they will feel seen, heard and less alone'
Maggie Dent, author of *Mothering Our Boys*

meltdown

Lauren Novak

HarperCollins*Publishers*

HarperCollins*Publishers*
Australia • Brazil • Canada • France • Germany • India • Italy • Japan
Mexico • Netherlands • New Zealand • Poland • Spain • Sweden
Switzerland • United Kingdom • United States of America

HarperCollins acknowledges the Traditional Custodians
of the lands upon which we live and work, and pays respect
to Elders past and present.

First published on Gadigal Country in Australia in 2026
by HarperCollins*Publishers* Australia Pty Limited
ABN 36 009 913 517
harpercollins.com.au

Copyright © Lauren Novak 2026

The right of Lauren Novak to be identified as the author of this work has been asserted by her in accordance with the *Copyright Act 1968*.

All rights reserved. Apart from any use as permitted under the *Copyright Act 1968*, no part may be reproduced, copied, scanned, stored in a retrieval system, recorded, or transmitted, in any form or by any means, without the prior written permission of the publisher. Without limiting the exclusive rights of any author, contributor, or the publisher of this publication, any unauthorised use of this publication to train generative artificial intelligence (AI) technologies is expressly prohibited. HarperCollins also exercises its rights under Article 4(3) of the Digital Single Market Directive 2019/790 and expressly reserves this publication from the text and data-mining exception.

HarperCollins*Publishers*
Macken House, 39/40 Mayor Street Upper
Dublin 1, D01 C9W8, Ireland

A catalogue record for this book is available from the National Library of Australia

ISBN 978 1 4607 6678 1 (paperback)
ISBN 978 1 4607 1802 5 (ebook)

Printed and bound in the UK using 100% Renewable Electricity at CPI Group (UK) Ltd

Cover design by Mietta Yans, HarperCollins Design Studio
Cover image by istockphoto.com
Author photograph by Ashleigh Dumont
Typeset in Sabon LT Std by Kirby Jones

Without limiting the exclusive rights of any author, contributor or the publisher of this publication, any unauthorised use of this publication to train generative artificial intelligence (AI) technologies is expressly prohibited. HarperCollins also exercise their rights under Article 4(3) of the Digital Single Market Directive 2019/790 and expressly reserve this publication from the text and data mining exception.

For my favourite kids in the whole wide world

Contents

Author's Note	xi
Foreword by Lael Stone	xiii
Introduction: My mum rage wake-up call	1
Part One: Mum Rage 101	**15**
It's a thing	17
Are all the other mums yelling this much?	28
A way to manage	41
What is anger?	49
What about the dads?	64
What if you're not the 'real' mum?	69
Part Two: Triggered	**73**
It's my hormones, Doc	75
Crying over lost sleep	84
Hangry mum	98
Pain in the … everything	108
Grief and loss	116

Part Three: Is This My Life Now?   **125**
We are forever changed   127
Mothering ain't what it used to be   134
Relentless provocation   149
More kids = more anger?   158

Part Four: It Feels Hard Because It Is   **165**
The self-care squeeze   167
Burning out   179
Crossing lines   189
Ghosts in the nursery   194
Being a Black mother in Australia   204

Part Five: The Juggle Is Real   **211**
Trying to make it work   213
The motherhood penalty   227
Default parent mode   232
Who said it would be 50/50?   245
Dude, where's my village?   255

Dad's right of reply   271
Epilogue: Am I still angry?   277
Acknowledgements   289
Endnotes   293

Author's Note

I pay my respects to the Kaurna people, the traditional owners of the land on which I live, wrote this book and raise my children.

The information in this book is based on my experience, recollections and research, and is not intended as professional or medical advice.

Some names and identifying details have been changed for privacy reasons.

I most commonly use the terms 'woman' and 'mother' because they are how I, and many of those I interviewed, identify; and because these words remind us that gender is at the heart of too many triggers for anger in motherhood. But not all mothers identify as women, and there are many ways to be a mother.

Please be aware this book deals with topics that can be triggering for some readers, including violence, suicide, suicidal ideation and pregnancy loss. If you need support, contact:

Lifeline – 13 11 14, lifeline.org.au
Beyond Blue – 1300 22 46 36, beyondblue.org.au
COPE (Centre of Perinatal Excellence) – 1300 740 398, cope.org.au
Gidget Foundation Australia – 1300 851 758, gidgetfoundation.org.au
PANDA (Perinatal Anxiety & Depression Australia) – 1300 726 306, panda.org.au
Postpartum Support International – postpartum.net
1800RESPECT (National Domestic Family and Sexual Violence Counselling Service) – 1800 737 732, 1800respect.org.au
13YARN (Aboriginal & Torres Strait Islander Crisis Support) – 13 92 76, 13yarn.org.au
Triple P – Positive Parenting Program – triplep-parenting.net.au

Foreword
By Lael Stone

I entered motherhood as a young woman who believed I could float through parenting with the same ease I'd navigated everything else in life. I was a relatively calm human who took life in their stride. Not much could faze me – until the morning my two-year-old wouldn't put his shoes on, and I completely lost it.

The shock was immense. This wasn't me. Where had this rage come from? In that moment, I came face to face with an anger I didn't know existed within me. Not just the frustration of dealing with a defiant toddler, but 27 years of repressed feelings that had finally found their breaking point. All those years of being the 'good girl' – of containing what society told me wasn't appropriate to feel or express – had culminated in this overwhelming eruption.

What I discovered through that experience, and what I've witnessed over 22 years of working with mothers, is that mum rage isn't a character flaw; it's a signal. It's our bodies and minds telling us that something fundamental needs attention. The lack of support, the absence of boundaries, the erasure of our own voices, and the impossible standards we're held to; it all builds up until it has nowhere else to go.

Lauren Novak understands this deeply. In *Meltdown*, she courageously explores the many threads that weave together to create maternal anger: the way we were raised, the current climate of impossible mothering expectations, the seismic shift in identity that motherhood brings and the overwhelming disparity in unpaid labour and responsibility that falls on mothers' shoulders. She examines the dance we do around 'who's doing it tougher', the guilt we carry for asking for help, and the tension that surfaces when we find ourselves competing with our partners for basic respites.

What makes this book so powerful is Lauren's willingness to share her own vulnerable journey through meltdown and finding a way to manage, combined with meticulous research and the stories of countless other mothers. She helps us understand that the feelings we've stored in our bodies, often for decades, need somewhere to go. When society fails to provide us with healthy ways to express anger, hurt and pain, it builds pressure that can eventually erupt, often directed at those we love most.

Through my own healing and in supporting other mothers, I've learned that one of the most crucial elements in reducing these meltdowns is having a safe place to be heard. When we bring experiences like mum rage into the light – instead of hiding them behind closed doors and thinking we're failing – something remarkable happens. They begin to lose their power over us.

Perhaps what's different now, from when I was a new mother 23 years ago, is that it's finally becoming safe enough to have these conversations openly. We're beginning to acknowledge that mothers are angry – and, frankly, it makes complete sense why we would be. The miracle is that we function as well as we do under such impossible circumstances.

When we stop hiding our struggles in shame, we create space for real change. Lauren's book is both a mirror and a map, reflecting our experiences back to us with compassion while showing us a way forward.

Every mother deserves to read this book. More than that, every mother deserves to be heard.

Introduction:
My mum rage wake-up call

It was a Friday night and our baby girl was finally asleep, cocooned in a bassinet next to the bed in our spare room. I spent the first six months of her life sleeping alongside her in that room, in an attempt to let her dad get some sleep in our main bedroom down the hallway. He's a tradie and, I hoped, would be less likely to fall off a roof or electrocute himself in an exhausted stupor if he wasn't woken quite as many times in the night as me.

By this particular Friday night, our daughter was one day shy of four months old and she had not been what you might call a 'good' sleeper. Her usual night-time routine involved refusing to settle for any decent stretch before midnight, then waking every hour or two for a feed until dawn. So, it was around midnight and there I was, lying in the spare bed next to her bassinet, trying to nod off while I had the chance. I'd left her dad downstairs after he fell asleep on the couch. I was just drifting off when I heard it. *Click.*

The bolt in the handle on our bedroom door had slipped into place with a sharp clunk that reverberated down the hallway. Much like being woken from deep sleep by the sound of a crying baby, it wrenched me back from the brink of unconsciousness. I sat bolt upright in bed, heart pounding, insides shaking. The rage was instantaneous. I threw off the quilt and lurched out of bed. So blinded was I by fury, I yanked open the door of the room my daughter and I were sleeping in, forgetting it might also wake her. I was so indignant, I don't think I cared. I slapped at the hallway light switch, flooding the corridor with bright white, and stomped down to our bedroom. When I burst through the door, I slammed on the lights in there too, just for good measure. 'Seriously, what the fuck?' I spat at the hump now ensconced under the covers. 'I had *just* fallen asleep!' I was properly yelling, having lost all regard for whether I might wake the baby (who, of course, slept through the whole thing).

I should pause here to point out that it hadn't even been a very loud noise. He hadn't run up the stairs shouting at the top of his lungs or anything. But you live in a house for a while and you get to know its sounds, and there had been no mistaking that click as the father of my child blithely let the door handle thud into place. We both know that if you slowly ease the door shut it won't make a sound. But (my sleep-deprived brain raged) that selfish man had paid no heed before wandering off to slumber peacefully in that enormous bed all on his own. And now here I was, *wiiiide* awake. The red mist had descended. I was so tired and so utterly outraged that my precious chance at sleep had been ruined, all bets were off. I had officially lost it.

Back to the bedroom. My partner sat up in bed. I think he might have told me to keep my voice down. Maybe he asked me what I was so worked up about. But I wasn't really listening. Nothing he could have said would have tempered

Introduction: My mum rage wake-up call

my fury in that moment. Throwing my arms in the air, I stomped out of the bedroom and back down the hallway. 'Well, I'm awake now, there's no way I'll be able to get back to sleep any time soon,' I yelled, shaking my head and flailing my limbs some more. What followed was more ranting about the other recent injustices I had endured, how I was doing all the heavy lifting raising this baby, sacrificing my body to grow, birth and feed her, how exhausted I was, how he clearly didn't understand or appreciate all this ... you get the gist. Absurdly, in the middle of my meltdown I even began opening cupboards and drawers. I figured that, given I was now upright, I might as well find and wrap the present I had bought to take to a first birthday party we were supposed to attend the following day. Or, more accurately, that day, as it was probably about 1 am by that point.

Looking back, I can see I overreacted. I can't remember how it ended – whether we had a screaming match and my partner retreated, leaving me to stew. Or whether, like he has done so many times since, he had been able to walk me back from the edge. I'm sure I cried. And at some point I must have gone back to bed. But, years later, what I can still remember – still feel in my body – is that searing anger. The boiling injustice I felt at being woken (to my mind) so inconsiderately when I had been sacrificing sleep, and everything else, for this child and her father for months. And I have felt it so many times since. Far more often than I ever thought I would when I first learned I would be a mum. Far more than anyone warned me.

There have been countless other times in the pitch black of night when I've let out a frustrated string of expletives because a baby has woken again after just 45 minutes. Or when I've yelled, 'Why won't you just go to sleep?' at a completely innocent and startled infant. Sometimes fear was at the heart of it, shamefully snapping at a preschooler because they wouldn't take medicine for a fever and I was sure they would overheat and die in the night. Other times it was envy, watching my partner head off to the footy with mates when I was too mentally exhausted to even think of what I would do if I had an afternoon to myself. There's been stomping off after having the same old fight about who changed the last pooey nappy and the general unfairness of the division of household labour. In fact, perceived unfairness is often at the root of my rage. (More on that later.)

It's not always an explosion; there's also plenty of the slow-burn kind of fuming that might happen when the other half disappears upstairs for 30 minutes right after arriving home from work. It can be seething muttering, bottled-up exasperation, tensed shoulders or grinding teeth. Sometimes it comes in the middle of the day, when the windows are open and the neighbours can hear me screaming at the kids who aren't listening, but in that moment I'm too far gone to stop out of embarrassment. Sometimes it's a sharp burst in the car when there are tiny feet kicking the back of my seat and a competition over who can make the most annoying noise the loudest. In every case, it is an inability to override the overwhelming impulse to release my own frustration.

Then, after the blow-up, there's the come-down. The guilt. The shame. The apologies. 'Mummy's sorry she yelled, sometimes she has big feelings too.' (Although far fewer apologies for the grown man I rage at – that always feels much harder.) At the end of each day, I promise myself I'll be better tomorrow. I've heard some parents refer to bedtime as a kind of do-over time, when all the day's parental failings can be forgiven with a cuddle and an extra book to read. A time when we are reminded of our child's unconditional love and that sinking feeling that we might not deserve it. Looking at their (finally) peaceful sleeping faces, round cheeks pressed flat against the mattress, their little chests rising and falling, I tell myself it will be fine in the morning. They'll forgive me. It might be relatively easy to wipe the slate clean when they're small, but it won't always.

Mum rage, as you may have heard it called, came as a surprise to me. I don't remember being yelled at as a child. It isn't the way I imagined parenting. However, in some families yelling, raging and worse is normal. It happens regularly, and it has been generational. But because it's something we don't feel safe talking about, it festers unnoticed behind closed doors and risks morphing into something dangerous. Even when it flares in public – when a mother smacks her kid in the supermarket, for instance – our usual response is to look away. How many of us would walk up and ask if she's okay, if she needs a hand? No one can help us if we aren't honest about how bad it is, but we're scared that if we're honest we'll be judged or punished. And this fear is far worse for mothers who already have the cards stacked against them because of where they live, what is (or isn't) in their bank account or the colour of their skin.

As parents, we don't talk about anger because it's not an acceptable emotion. We tell ourselves that we should be able to control it. If we can't, there's something wrong with us. We're a bad example to our children, even a danger to them. And there is an implicit judgement that to be angry is to be ungrateful. If our children are so wanted and so cherished then to be angry at them, or because of them, brings into question whether we really appreciate them. Whether we deserve them. If we can't handle the stresses of being a parent then why did we choose to be one? If we can't put our own selfish emotions aside then why do we deserve the gift of children when so many others would kill for what we have? So the guilt and shame and fear that bubble around our mum rage stop us from talking about it, from confiding in anyone – until it simply boils over.

The truth is mum rage happens to most of us. Even if no one warns us, it is more common than we think. And the first step to getting on top of it is to start talking about it. I've spent more than a year examining what triggers my mum rage and what actually helps to manage it. (Spoiler alert: it's not taking a deep breath.) If you're reading this book then you're probably looking for these answers too. I can't promise that by the time you turn the final page you'll be a Zen guru with the patience of Mary Poppins. But, if nothing else, you will know that you are not alone, and that feeling this way does not make you a bad mum. And you'll have some ideas about how to recognise and manage your triggers, or help others to.

It can be almost impossible to step back from the madness when you're in it but, by taking off my mum hat and putting on the one I wear in my day job as a journalist, I was able to gain a semblance of perspective that showed me there were key factors at play. The sleep deprivation that comes with parenting little ones decimates our ability to control many basic functions, including regulating our mood. 'Hangry' (that desperate combination of hungry and angry) is taken to the extreme when you're trapped under a sleeping baby without snacks in reach, stuck in the car driving from soccer practice to a dance recital or just too busy or stressed to eat properly. Hormones of course play a part in the months (and, I've now learned, years) after giving birth, but these are too often blamed as the only reason for our rage. Expectations of mothers have changed over the decades. Far more families are juggling work and kids because of the rising cost of living. And way more of us than are willing to admit are furious at our spouses for possessing useless nipples and somehow being able to hold on to their old life while we barely make it through the transition to motherhood.

The underlying factors that fuel this kind of anger differ widely depending on which mum we're talking about. What about the mums managing pain or chronic illness? Mums who face racism and discrimination, or whose children do? Parents and carers of children with disability, complex needs or trauma? The families fighting to stay above the poverty line? Some of these factors are within our individual control. Many are part of a bigger system that will take more to change than scheduling a half-hour of self-care journalling while grandma takes bubs for a walk around the block.

For so long I was too agitated to do any of the things that everyone told me would calm me. I was too agitated to meditate. I was too agitated to learn new parenting skills or scripts. I was too agitated to even ask for help. It became clear that to get to a place where I could do these things, I was going to have to change some of the basics first. I needed more sleep. I needed to move my body. And I needed more time on my own. To get any of that, I needed more support. In the coming chapters, I'll take you through some of the most common factors contributing to mum rage in homes across Australia – and the world. I'll share with you what I've learned from experts and other families, and what has ultimately helped me.

I asked how anger works in our brains and bodies, and how things like lack of sleep, poor nutrition, hunger and pain affect our ability to manage our mood. I wanted to know if more kids mean more anger, if it is harder to be a mum today than 50 years ago, and how our own childhoods influence our parenting. I delved into the data on who does what in Australian households, who bears the mental load, and how mums face hurdles whether they stay at home or return to paid work. And I came to understand how losing our sense of self in motherhood can be devastating. Along the way, I gathered advice and consolidated my own thoughts on what each of us can do and what needs to change on a grander scale.

Because we must do something. Perinatal mental health issues like depression and anxiety affect one in five new mums, and one in ten dads.[1] A 2019 report by PricewaterhouseCoopers found these issues are costing Australia $877 million a year in lost productivity, health system demand and generational mental ill health.[2] And did you know suicide is among the top causes of maternal death.[3] In the state of Victoria, ten mothers died by suicide in the five years to 2017.⁴ However, these figures only capture the period of pregnancy up to 42 days after birth. Other data, which extended to one year postpartum, shows that 15 mothers in New South Wales died by suicide in the six years to 2007,⁵ and there were three suicides by mothers in South Australia in 2022 alone.⁶ As a journalist I have reported on the suicides of at least five mothers who were further into parenting before the despair set in. We might think of sadness or hopelessness as the overriding emotions in these cases, but anger is undoubtedly boiling in the mix too.

We need to start talking more and asking for more help. A 2024 survey of 5000 Australians, commissioned by Beyond Blue, found just over a quarter of people who experienced a mental health challenge in the past year did not seek *any* support. And half of those who sought professional help waited until they were 'very distressed' or 'extremely distressed'. Cost and availability were major deterrents and more than one in five were kept quiet by shame.⁷ Mum rage is not a diagnosable mental illness or condition, but it can be a warning sign of one. It wasn't until doing research for this book that I learned irritability and anger could be symptoms of depression, anxiety or crippling hormonal conditions.

In some scenarios, anger left unchecked can escalate and lead to harm to children. There are lines that we, as a society, draw when anger crosses over into abuse. There are parents who intentionally beat their children, lock them up, deprive them or berate and humiliate them without remorse. But the lines blur around the edges. Surprisingly large numbers of parents still believe smacking is a useful disciplinary tool despite a growing body of evidence that shows it does long-term damage to children. How do we determine when yelling crosses the line into verbal, emotional or psychological abuse, or when our inability to regulate our own emotions tips from having a bad day to putting our children at risk? And how much is kept hidden behind closed doors because of shame about falling on the wrong side of these lines?

I have spent the past two decades as a journalist grappling with many of these issues, but always through the telling of other people's stories. To be this public about my own life is an unnatural and uncomfortable pivot. It feels risky to reveal so much. People who know me might never look at me the same way after reading my confessions. (Others might say they had an inkling ...) So why is it worth the risk? Because, frankly, it shouldn't *be* a risk. Admitting we are not okay should not be risky. Asking for help should not be risky. The real risk is if this rage goes unaddressed. The real risk is in *not* being honest with ourselves – and with others.

I know some will argue that writing this book is a self-indulgent attempt to absolve my guilt or pardon myself. There will be plenty who label me a terrible mum based on what they read in these pages. They will say I don't deserve my children, that I'm self-centred and not up to the job. It's nothing I haven't heard before, rattling around in my own brain. And *that* is the reason I've written this book. Because there are too many mums beating themselves up for something that is far, far more common than we are led to believe. We love our children *so* much and we don't *want* to be this angry. I always wanted to be a mum, and I am stopped in my tracks each day by moments of heart-cracking joy at watching my children grow, learn and love me back. I break into a full-face smile every time my son asks me if I'm driving under 'the speed lemon' or my daughter tells me she's 'writing a book' at school. I am living out a lifelong dream every time I get to hold their hands as we walk down the road. And the weight of a little body nestled into my lap for a cuddle might just be the best feeling in the world.

But what I have learned is that the angry moments are, in many cases, a normal reaction to the circumstances we can face: the steep learning curve of new motherhood, the hormonal rollercoaster, the lack of a village to support us, the juggle with paid work, the loss of our identity, and society's totally unachievable expectations of modern mothers. The problems come when we act on the anger in uncontrolled ways. When anger becomes aggression. The occasional outburst morphs into constant irritability, an ever-present dark cloud over our head, overwhelming rage or eventual burnout. Then we fall into a shame spiral about it all so that the problems stay behind closed doors, where they can grow ever more dangerous. This book is not about rationalising or absolution. It is not about normalising child abuse or harmful expressions of rage. But it is about acknowledging that this is how we can feel, and giving us the knowledge to reflect on why. It's a flare into the night sky, illuminating a struggling mum in the rowboat below. It's a call for us to confide in one another, and ask for help, before we are too far out at sea.

Not all mums will grapple with these feelings or feel them with the same intensity. The spectrum of human temperament is a wide one and we all exist at different points along it. There were some mums I spoke to who said mum rage just didn't affect them. A few said the anger flared but they didn't feel it was a problem. But far more of us are suffering, or simmering, in silence than anyone realises. In fact, one psychologist I spoke to said that 'every single mother' she sees has experienced anger towards their child at some point. In a survey I ran of 200 mums (my 'Angry Mums Club', as I've come to call them), just *four* said they had never experienced anger in motherhood (although three of those conceded to 'frustration'). When it came down to it, I realised my anger was affecting not just me and how I felt about myself as a mum, but also my kids, my partner, my parents, my health. Everyone has bad moments or bad days, but this horrible mood was rearing its ugly head every day. I knew I couldn't just ride it out because it's not only babies or toddlers that give parents the shits, and I imagine the teenage years will be just as testing (swapping out postnatal struggles for perimenopausal ones). I needed to find a better way for our family, but also to get real with those at the start of their parenting journey about what could be coming down the pipeline, and how they might handle it better.

Beneath my fear of being judged for being a bad mum lies a much stronger motivation for writing a book like this. One of my greatest worries is that my angry mum moments will seep into my children. Right now, they are young, forgiving and forgetful, but already I see glimpses of my meltdowns in them. At their 21st birthday parties we will laugh about how our two-year-old son learned to yell 'fustated' at the top of his lungs when I had an outburst. (At least he was learning the emotional intelligence to name his feelings, right?) Or how our daughter picked up the phrase 'fucky sake' from her mother. But it isn't funny when I think about what they must see when I'm yelling, wild-eyed, at one of them to get back into bed after they've woken me up for the fourth time that night.

As I learned more about why I feel this way, I began to worry about whether my kids would struggle like me in adulthood. If they became parents, would the societal expectations of mums still be as infuriating? Would the balance of parenting still feel so unfair? Would the whole thing still be shrouded in secrecy? This intergenerational concern surfaced during my research one day in, of all places, a children's movie (yes, it was research). I'd heard a mum confess on a podcast that during her rage moments, her children compared her to the giant pandas in the heartwarming but unnervingly relatable Disney Pixar film *Turning Red*.[8] The animated tale centres on 13-year-old Meilin Lee, who is grappling with her first menstrual cycle, and discovering that a generational family curse means she will also now turn into a giant red panda whenever she is overcome with emotion. In one scene, the young girl explodes into panda mode when she is embarrassed by her mother showing up to her school waving sanitary pads in front of her classmates. She's able to get a handle on things when she realises that taking deep breaths to calm down reverses the transformation. (Glad it works for some!) The culmination of the film is a grand battle when all the women of the family release their moody pandas and a huge emotional fight erupts.

I don't want my rage to be intergenerational. For too many families it already is. Mum rage is no joke, and telling us it is just part of the parenting deal won't cut it. When I began writing this book, I wasn't sure if I could rein in the anger for myself, let alone tell anyone else how to do so. All I knew was it was going to take more than a few deep breaths.

Part One

Mum Rage 101

It's a thing

If it was the click of a door that awoke me to my mum rage, it was toilet training that broke me. The relentless, unpredictable, hypervigilant, frustrating 'when will this end' rollercoaster of toilet training. For some kids it just happens: three days of running around in the nude and they're potty pros. This was not the case for our kids and it did not sit well with my A-type perfectionist multitasking personality. I cannot tell you how many hours I sat on the tiled floors of toilets all over town, how many creative incentives I conjured, how many YouTube videos I played featuring cartoon characters singing about wees and poos. One step forward, two steps back … for months on end.

Many, many times I calmly cleaned up accidents, put pint-sized undies in the washing machine and gave encouragement for next time. It wasn't the accidents that bothered me, they happen. It was the wind-up. More times than I'd like to admit, I was impatient for it to be over, hurrying a fidgety toddler. You can lead them to the dunny but you can't make them do their business. One day, it was just all too much. I was running on too little sleep, I'd sat down for what felt like the first time all day, and just as my bum hit the couch: 'Muuuuuum'. The tone told me all I needed to know. It was toilet time.

Cue 15 minutes of faffing, on and off the loo, promising chocolates, stickers, anything ... and all of a sudden I was overcome with rage. I couldn't suppress it any longer. 'That's it, I'm sick of this!' I screeched, before stomping upstairs to sit on my bed and angry cry, leaving a bewildered little person and their dad downstairs. That was when I realised I needed help. All the things that were combining and building to make me feel this way were getting the better of me, and I could see no relief in sight. This wasn't the kind of parent I wanted to be. The occasional outburst had turned into a constant baseline of irritation. I had a short fuse and zero patience. I was on edge, worn down and burned out. I was trying the things we're told to do – deep breaths, counting, taking a moment before you react – but these tools were feeble in the face of the relentless onslaught of parenting.

An initial search of the internet for help was not helpful. It yielded mum rage memes about it being 'that time of the month' or mummy forgetting to take her 'happy pills'. The government-funded parenting websites popped up with their obvious dot points about trying to get enough sleep or putting the baby down in the cot and walking away if you're feeling like you might shake them. (But what about when they are old enough to follow you?!) Then there were the endless listicles like 'Why am I an angry mom? 7 common anger triggers and how to deal with them', which helpfully suggested waking up before everyone else in the house to 'have some time alone in peace'.[1] I was already setting my alarm for 5 am on workdays to try to do a half-hour of yoga in the pitch dark, without making any noise, because it was the only chance I might get. But our kids have always been early risers and inevitably most days one, if not both, of them was awake minutes after I rolled out my yoga mat.

Don't get me wrong, I'm not angry all the time. I take so much joy in my sweet, cheeky, clever kids every day. They are *the* best things in my life. For as long as I can remember I wanted children, and my heart swells to bursting when my unbelievably healthy and mostly happy kids plant slobbery kisses on my face (even when that slobber delivers the Covid virus directly into my system). I am obsessed with their implausibly soft cheeks and little chipmunk voices. There is no better sound than when they dissolve into fits of giggles over something silly, reminding me to see the lighter side. Every day, I look at my tiny humans and marvel at how incredible they are, these smart little sponges soaking up the world around them. And I love and appreciate the man with whom I've chosen to make this life and raise these kids. They have his curls, and I hope they will inherit his patience, self-belief, imaginative streak and sense of fun too. But parenting has forever changed our relationship, and it takes more work than ever to keep choosing each other, day after (long and trying) day. I'm a lot angrier, a lot more often, than I was before we had kids. More than I could have imagined I would be as a mum. More than I want to be and certainly more than anyone told me I might be!

This was not part of the curriculum in antenatal classes. None of our friends who lurched into parenthood before us confessed to midnight screaming matches or uncontrolled outbursts at the relentlessness of it all. Maybe they're just better people. I certainly feel like a bad mum every time it gets the better of me. But, more likely, no one talked to us about this because it's difficult to admit. Anger is not an emotion you're *supposed* to feel towards your children, or your partner. And if you do, you're supposed to feel guilty about it. So it's no surprise in hindsight that these kinds of stories weren't shared alongside the warnings about sleep deprivation, changes to your body or the complete loss of a social life. Sure, they told us kids can be frustrating. We heard tales of preschoolers ignoring parents' repeated requests to put on shoes, or mortifying meltdowns in the supermarket over a chocolate bar. But these stories were usually relayed in jest.

Like so many things about parenting, there is an argument that you can't really understand mum rage until you experience it. I remember one friend who entered motherhood ahead of me texting a photo of her toddler having a full-blown tantrum, face-down on the bathroom tiles. 'I wouldn't let him drink the shower water off the floor,' she explained matter-of-factly. I laughed at the time. But now I know exactly how irrational and infuriating that situation would have been. I also know that it could have come at the end of a long string of irrational and infuriating toddler tantrums, after a night of little sleep, while she may have been recovering from mastitis or worrying about returning to work.

Few parents are open about the depth of their fury – and using the word 'angry' is still taboo. I'd certainly never heard a mum publicly acknowledge feeling this way before it happened to me. So when I felt it, I felt ashamed. I figured it had to be a fault in me. I wasn't able to control my anger. I was a bad mum.

As I waited to bring my much-longed-for first child into the world, I had been more prepared to be sad or a nervous wreck. Stigma remains around postnatal depression and anxiety, but we do talk more openly now about the possibility of both with expecting parents. My mother had warned me about the 'baby blues', so when they hit about two days after our daughter was born, I was overwhelmed but not ashamed.

The kind of rage that emerged for me later in motherhood was not something anyone had given me a heads-up about. Instead, like so many revelations in the modern age, I had a lightbulb moment through social media. I stumbled across a video posted to Instagram by American nurse and mother of five Karrie Locher.[2] The gist of it: postpartum rage, it's a thing. I came across that video while sitting in the dark, back in our spare room, nursing our son to sleep almost two years after my blow-up about being woken by the click of a door handle. Two years (and another baby) later and I was still experiencing that rage. It hadn't eased over time. I hadn't 'got on top of it'. I hadn't grown out of it. It still simmered and then boiled over. But at least now I knew I wasn't the only mum in the world who felt this way.

Seeing it discussed on social media was a gateway to talking about it in the real world. Tentatively, I began broaching it with other mums. 'Do you, like, sometimes get a bit frustrated ... and maybe, like, yell?'

'Oh my gosh, yes,' came the replies. 'All the time! I was so angry the other night I slammed the door and woke the baby up!'

Once I started talking about it with other mums (rather than yelling about it to my kids and partner), I found I couldn't stop – and it turned out almost every other mum around me was raging too. It was like opening a secret door to a speakeasy where, in whispered tones, parents would confess to the truth of their hidden emotions. 'In the moment I am so mad and frustrated. Almost immediately afterwards I feel so guilty and upset at myself,' one mum of two in her 30s confided. Another, with five kids, feels 'completely justified during' an outburst and 'full of regret and shame afterwards. It's like a switch is flicked and all of a sudden I can't contain it anymore,' she told me. 'It's often the build-up of lots of little things that I think I can handle and one more pushing me over the edge. I can't always remember it clearly afterwards.' (Well, that sounds familiar ...)

Mums today are often overstimulated, under-supported, disconnected, constantly comparing and feeling guilty. Many of us have come to parenting after establishing independent careers and living autonomous, productive lives where we called the shots. Then, overnight, we had to surrender to the demands of a small human who relied on us for survival but cared not that we used to be highly regarded in our paid job or might like to visit the toilet alone once in a while. All the things we are told to do to preserve our mental health – exercise, eat well, get enough sleep, socialise – seem utterly impossible. But mums of my generation, millennials, in particular, seem to have been conditioned to believe we should be able to have and do it all. We're failing if we can't, or lacking ambition if we don't want to. We're also part of a generation that was raised to expect equality, at work and at home, but that utopia hasn't quite arrived. On top of all that, the life-altering transition into parenthood occurred for many of us in the middle of the worldwide COVID-19 pandemic, during which an unpredictable and deadly virus spread unabated across the globe, further isolating us and ushering in an era of complete paranoia and hypervigilance. No wonder we're on edge.

To get a better understanding of how other mums were feeling, and what was happening in their homes, I created an anonymous online survey. About 200 people responded. I refer to them as members of my Angry Mums Club, although we don't have meetings or anything. In fact, I've never met many of them. I can't tell you how old they are, how many kids they have or much about their cultural background because I didn't want to ask any identifying questions that might put them off answering completely honestly. But they include single and partnered, straight and queer mums of one or many kids from European, Asian, Aboriginal and other backgrounds, living around Australia and overseas. For the vast majority in the Angry Mums Club, their first experience of a 'mum meltdown' was followed by feelings of guilt (85 per cent), shame (70 per cent), remorse (65 per cent) and anxiety (50 per cent). During outbursts, half said they feel 'out of control' and one in five reported having a kind of 'out of body' experience. Asked to rate the intensity of their mum rage out of ten, more than half gave a rating of between six and ten. Notably, when asked how often they felt irritated in their role as a mother, not a single one said 'never'. *Not one.* Almost half felt irritated multiple times a day. Almost two in every five felt angry multiple times a week and nearly a third had at least weekly episodes of downright rage.

For me, it usually surfaces as yelling and (shamefully) swearing. Among the Angry Mums Club, nearly 60 per cent had screamed (the most common expression) at their child and 45 per cent had told their child to 'go away'. About two in every five had slammed a door in anger and told a child to 'shut up'. A third had sworn at a youngster. A quarter had smacked or hit their kid. Others admitted to covering their ears, kicking or throwing things in frustration and walking away from children having tantrums in public. About half also harboured desires to run away or have an extended period of time alone. (One mum confessed to a community nurse that she imagined being injured in a car accident just so she could 'have a break'. Another said she sometimes had suicidal thoughts when the anger was 'really bad'.) Despite how common it clearly is to feel (and act) this way, one in five in the Club had never spoken to another mother about these feelings. Less than half had sought the help of any kind of professional, such as a GP, psychologist or helpline counsellor. Guilt and shame kept most quiet, along with the fear of being judged. Most mums were taken by surprise when the anger emerged. Three-quarters said either no one had warned them about mum rage or they couldn't remember it being raised. Only 12 mums said they were warned seriously.

When I asked what the Angry Mums Club members wanted most from a book like this, the overwhelming majority said they just wanted to know they weren't alone. 'Solidarity', one wrote simply. 'Honesty', wrote another. One pleaded for 'stories of other mums' anger so I don't feel so alone [and] so bad about myself'.

So I hope they – and you – will feel a bit better to hear that, in one of my first interviews for this book, I asked clinical and counselling psychologist Annabel Hales how common anger in motherhood is, and her reply came quickly and confidently:

'Very common. I would say every single mother I have come across has had an experience of anger and reactivity towards their child. They've had a moment where they have said something, done something, that they're not proud of. The master story [of motherhood] is "How privileged am I, how wonderful are children, these gorgeous little creatures." But the story behind the story is grief, powerlessness, lack of control, exhaustion and then the shame cycle around that. "I'm just a bad mum. There's something wrong with me. I'm going to screw up my child."'

Hales has felt it herself. Over video chat she told me of a time when her baby son was crying and Hales had to put him down in his cot and go to the other end of the house. As she recounted the story, I could see her hands clench into fists at the bottom of the laptop screen. 'My body remembers that,' she said, looking at her hands. Another time she was driving with her son screaming in his car seat. Feeling stuck and at a loss, she could still remember the 'white, white-hot rage'. Mums who feel this way are 'having a physiological response that needs to be taken care of', Hales said, and it needs to be 'placed within biological and historical contexts'.

This is part of what motherhood studies sociologist Sophie Brock has dedicated her career to doing. A single mum of one in Sydney, Dr Brock developed the Fish Tank model of motherhood to illustrate how we mums (the fish) are shaped by society (the tank) and its expectations (the water) about how we mother (or how we swim). Most of us come into motherhood not knowing what's swirling in the water around us, it's just always been there. So one of Dr Brock's go-to pieces of advice is to encourage us fish to pull out a big black texta and start scribbling on the glass walls of our tank 'all the rules of what it means to be a good mum'. When we can see the 'shoulds' of motherhood more clearly, we can understand that our feelings of frustration and anger can be a 'reasonable response to the circumstances we're put in and the pressure we're under'. Feeling that we're failing to live up to these expectations leads us into what Dr Brock terms the 'anger–guilt trap'. We beat ourselves up for not being good enough, we get frustrated and angry, then we feel guilty about getting angry, so we double down on trying to meet those unmeetable standards …. aaaaand round we go again. Among the Angry Mums Club, three-quarters said they felt guilty after an outburst. About a third would berate themselves, while a quarter would overcompensate by trying to be extra calm or positive afterwards.

Many in the Club also wanted to know if it was just us or if mums were this angry 50 years ago. We'll look in more detail later at how motherhood has changed over the decades, but modern mums are not outliers. Back in 1976, poet, author and mother Adrienne Rich published *Of Woman Born: Motherhood as experience and institution*. When I finally cracked open this book in 2024 it was a revelation. Rich, whose children were born in the 1950s, wrote of finding common ground with other mothers 'in an unacceptable but undeniable anger'. She talked of 'held-in rage' and 'a tangle of irritations deepening to anger'.[3] Fast-forward two decades and, in 1996, sociologist Sharon Hays gave voice in her book *The Cultural Contradictions of Motherhood* to the frustrations of American mothers struggling to raise children, do everything at home and often work for pay as well. She conducted in-depth interviews with a sample of American mums and found many were 'left feeling pressed for time, a little guilty, a bit inadequate and somewhat ambivalent about their position'.[4] A couple of years later, in 1998, prolific American writer Anne Lamott detailed, with dry humour and surprising honesty, the tedium of parenting that drives many of us to rage. In an article for news and opinion website Salon titled 'Mother rage: theory and practice', she recounted the bedtime battle that prompted her to threaten the safety of her son's pets, and the time she screamed at him 'with such rage' because he was ignoring her that it was as if he'd tried to set her bed on fire.[5] The more I read, the more I discovered that mum rage was not new – it was just new to me.

These women had long been trying to warn us. How had I not heard them? I'm a reader. I'm a journalist. I was raised in a feminist household. Still, I hadn't found their missives before I needed them. The reality is none of us go looking for angry mum stories before we have kids because we don't realise we'll need them. When we're pregnant, Heidi Murkoff's cult classic *What to Expect When You're Expecting* or Kaz Cooke's quirky *Up the Duff* are more likely to be on our bedside table, as we obsess over which fruit our fetus resembles that week or try to decide on a birth plan. But the truth is out there. Mum rage is a thing.

Are all the other mums yelling this much?

The simple answer is 'yes'. While there is still a strong taboo around talking about mum rage, don't believe for one second that you are the only one experiencing it. You've already heard parts of my story and seen the almost uniform response from the Angry Mums Club. In fact, among its 200 members only 10 per cent said they never yelled. Almost a third yelled at their kids multiple times a week. The 2024 National Parenting Pulse Survey of more than 8300 Australian parents found eight in ten yelled or raised their voice at their kids at some point. Almost half did so at least weekly, and 14 per cent yelled at least once *every* day.[1]

A quick search of conversations on social media yields more proof of the ubiquity of frustration and anger in parenthood. This is a selection of what just a few mums said on the question-and-answer platform Reddit:

> 'I feel like my mum rage is crushing my chest. I want to pick my son up and shake him.'
> 'My son says mommy 100000000xs and I want to stab my eardrums so I never have to hear it again.'
> 'The rage that would course through me was frightening.'

'Sometimes I snarl and I pull my own hair and smack myself. Sometimes I'll scream into my pillows. I feel so angry.'

'I am a freaking monster. Like unbelievably short-fused and so mean. This is not me.'[2]

If you asked an expectant first-time mother today if she could imagine herself typing words like this in the months or years ahead, she would probably look at you in wide-eyed horror. But we are starting to glimpse more representations of these kinds of mums in popular culture. In the 2021 film *The Lost Daughter*, we see the character Leda Caruso struggle with the overstimulation and restriction of parenting, eventually abandoning her daughters and their father. In the dark comedy TV series *Breeders*, fictional British mum Ally Worsley declares – after letting fly in a menopause-induced fit of rage – 'I am not a bad mother, I am a good mother at the end of her rope.' In Jessamine Chan's novel *The School for Good Mothers*, sleep-deprived Frida Liu leaves her toddler daughter home alone to escape the relentlessness of parenting and ends up in a futuristic re-education centre for bad mums. And there's Rachel Yoder's novel *Nightbitch*, whose central character of the same name – a mother of a toddler son – asks readers, 'How could you *not* be pissed after having a baby?'[3]

More women are confessing to their real-life rage too, like journalist and author Lucy Jones, who recounts, in her 2023 book *Matrescence: On the metamorphosis of pregnancy, childbirth and motherhood,* how she deliberately smashed coffee mugs on her concrete back patio after a particularly frustrating outing with her baby.[4] Or academic and author

Nancy Reddy, who admits in her 2025 book *The Good Mother Myth: Unlearning our bad ideas about how to be a good mom* that she was so infuriated by difficulties pumping breastmilk that she bit into a baby bottle.[5] The first of these brave confessions that I stumbled upon (in early 2023, when my youngest child was not quite two) was a 2019 *New York Times* essay by Minna Dubin. The California-based mother of two's piece 'The rage mothers don't talk about' reflected what I had been feeling far more honestly than I had seen anywhere else. 'In this red place, I yell at my son so hard my voice becomes a growl,' Dubin wrote.[6] She told me later she had been nervous to share but was inundated by 'thank yous' and 'me toos' from readers. The response to that piece, and a follow-up during the COVID-19 pandemic when American mothers gathered in fields to scream to release their rage, led Dubin to write *Mom Rage: The everyday crisis of modern motherhood*, released towards the end of 2023.[7]

After reading it (in one sitting) I briefly wondered if I should even bother writing a book on anger in motherhood – it appeared this had already been done. But when I plucked up the courage to ask Dubin if she would speak to me for this project, she reassured me that more voices are always welcome in the conversation – which has started to shift. 'The phrase "mum rage", it's all over the place now,' she said. 'The idea of maternal ambivalence, maternal anger, maternal regret ... all of that is swirling in the zeitgeist.' But people are still 'very, very uncomfortable to this day with the idea of a mother being furious', Dubin said. When it comes to voicing the depth of rage some of us feel, 'it's like a live wire and nobody wants to touch it'. And if they do, it's usually to criticise. Dubin told me it was 'very scary' to publish how she felt, and she took 'a lot of precautions to protect myself and my family because I was terrified of how the world would respond. I got emails, I got messages ... they said, still say, things like "You shouldn't be a mother", "You're mentally ill". They're awful, I try and delete them before I read them.' Although, Dubin added, the trolls are buried by the deluge of stories from women all over the world who relate to the rage.

International research supports this. Back in 2002, the authors of a New York study titled 'Anger after childbirth: an overlooked reaction to postpartum stressors' surveyed 163 middle- to upper-class women when pregnant and again at least a month after birth. They found a third reported 'moderate to high levels of anger'. At least two in five of those angry new mums had not described themselves as particularly angry prior to having kids.[8] In a 2006 study of 204 mothers who had been referred to mother–baby services in New Zealand and England, more than a quarter exhibited at least some anger towards their baby, and 8 per cent were severely angry.[9] More recently, Canadian researchers interviewed 18 mothers for the 2022 paper 'Seeing red: a grounded theory study of women's anger after childbirth'. All but one had experienced intense anger. (Half were first-time mums.) They described stomping, slamming doors, breaking or throwing things, punching pillows or screaming into them, clenching their fists and gritting their teeth. They cried, sent children to time-out and had heated arguments with partners. Often these women tried to keep their anger to themselves, to appear like they were coping.[10]

When I put out a call for raging mums Down Under, one of the first to reply was Eleni, a 34-year-old mother of two living in Auckland, New Zealand. A former teacher, now stay-at-home mum, Eleni had a daughter and son 20 months apart. She told me she was warned about depression, but not anger. At first, she thought she was irritable just from a lack of sleep. As time went on, she began to feel 'touched out', avoiding both her children, aged five and three by the time she got in touch with me, and her husband. 'I felt completely out of control with my own emotions,' Eleni wrote in her courageously honest response to my questions. 'It felt relentless and like no matter how I tried to regulate my emotions, nothing worked. I'd find myself reacting by yelling and shutting myself in the bedroom. The rage or blow-ups I had were definitely triggered by touch, when my children climbed on me or my partner would cuddle me. I couldn't cope with the feeling of my space being taken away. The guilt was immense and I couldn't believe I was such a bad parent that I didn't want to touch my children. My husband didn't understand ... and I got the impression he felt rejected and lonely.'

After the birth of her son, Eleni visited her GP and confided she had yelled at her toddler a few times. She said the doctor told her she was 'a good parent' because she felt bad about it when she yelled. 'I wasn't given any help or advice with the situation but simply told my feelings of guilt and inadequacy were enough to make me a good parent.' A fear of being judged, or even having her children removed, prevented Eleni from confiding in anyone else. 'Sometimes in conversations with close friends I've said that I'm feeling "over the kids" or that they were driving me crazy [but] I've never had an explicit conversation about feeling anger, rage or anything more than frustration and overwhelm,' she said. 'I think deep down I've been afraid people wouldn't trust me if I couldn't manage my emotions all the time. Or they might be concerned about the children's wellbeing and report me for emotional abuse if I admitted I'd lost my cool and yelled at them too many times.'

As I read Eleni's story, I felt as if it could be my own. A girl and a boy, 20 months apart. Sleep deprivation. Feeling touched out, rageful then guilty and fearful. Eleni has struggled with asking for help too. 'I have people I can ask to take the kids if I need a break ... but I feel guilty for handing my kids over to someone else and then they have expectations of me, or they tell me how to use my time, which dredges up more guilt and obligation.'

Eleni and I are not alone. About a third of Angry Mums Club members felt guilty multiple times a week about feeling frustration or rage. Only ten mums said they never felt guilt about feeling, or expressing, their anger. Perth mother of three Jing told me how she would get her three kids into bed at night and then 'just look at their quiet, sleeping bodies and feel tremendous guilt every night for how I had treated them during the day'. The 2024 National Parenting Pulse Survey, conducted by University of Queensland academics, found a sad (but not surprising) 30 per cent of mums felt guilty at least once a day – and it was more common among mums of children aged under five. (Yep, that checks out.) Guilt is important in letting us know when we've crossed a line in our parenting, prompting us to check back in with our values. But the survey authors warn it can be problematic if it is 'persistent, intense and does not lead the parent to make any change'.[11]

Aside from the guilt spiral, what else contributes to mum rage? Angry Mums Club members overwhelmingly nominated lack of sleep (80 per cent) as the top factor that contributed to their level of background irritability, frustration and anger. After that it was an extremely tight race between feeling like the parenting load was not shared equally with a spouse or co-parent, keeping up with household tasks, worries about parental responsibilities, the relentlessness of parenting and hormone fluctuations (which ranged from 53 to 57 per cent). In the moment of an outburst, the biggest trigger was feeling that a child wasn't listening (65 per cent), followed by being overstimulated by the noise and demands of parenting (53 per cent) and having to repeat instructions to a child (49 per cent).

'Put your shoes on, honey … Please put your shoes on … One, two, three … PUT ON YOUR DAMN SHOES!'

We've all been there, right?

More rigorous surveys than mine have uncovered similar patterns. A 2018 poll by the Royal Children's Hospital Melbourne found a quarter of parents felt stressed by their child's behaviour every day. Almost half felt they became impatient too quickly and a third conceded they often lost their temper and later felt guilty. Asked how they had disciplined their child in the previous month, 61 per cent said they had shouted or yelled. A third had made their child 'feel bad to teach them a lesson'. Almost a quarter had threatened physical discipline, such as smacking, and 17 per cent had followed through.[12]

In 2021, Australia's Centre of Perinatal Excellence (COPE) conducted federally funded research to develop an awareness campaign about the realities of parenting. Almost 1900 mums and dads took a survey and more than 600 provided detailed comments. Among them were admissions of unexpected anger, followed by 'immense feelings of guilt and shame'. One woman spoke of having 'a very short fuse and no precursor to [an] outburst'. Another resented her husband for how 'little his life had changed' and her 'endlessly unsettled baby'.

Many people said the feelings of rage were 'not something they ever associated with having a baby' nor was anger raised by health professionals. These feelings were compounded for families who had gone through assisted reproduction or IVF, who felt guilty about their rage because of how much they had longed for a child and what they had been through to have one.[13]

Ariane Beeston was on the team that conducted the research. She knows a thing or two about how difficult it can be to express how we're feeling postpartum. Beeston's 2024 memoir, *Because I'm Not Myself, You See*, charts her experience of postnatal depression and psychosis. In it she mentions having flashes of rage, including throwing a plate on the ground during an argument with her husband. When we spoke via video call on a chilly day in her hometown of Melbourne, Beeston told me her rage moments were mostly related to adjusting to the cocktail of medications she was prescribed to manage her illness. But she knows how these feelings can emerge in motherhood. She started her career as a caseworker and psychologist in the New South Wales child protection system and, while working in the hotline call centre, Beeston took calls from people reporting parents who had shaken their babies, often when sleep deprived and in the face of incessant crying. It wasn't until she became a mother that she had a 'profound moment of realisation' about how a parent could 'snap' like that. Beeston later worked as a parenting journalist before joining COPE, where she is the communications manager.

She told me that the page on the COPE website explaining maternal rage is one of its most visited. 'We expect to be sleep deprived but we don't expect to necessarily be pissed off and full of rage,' she said. 'It does feel like anger is the last taboo. Women are much more comfortable talking about postnatal depression, anxiety, even psychosis. But when it comes to rage, it really goes against everything that we assume a mother should be. They might say they're burned out, or struggling with the mental load, or other language, but it's still difficult to say, "I'm just really pissed off."'

The COPE research led to an awareness campaign titled The Truth. But if mum rage is, indeed, part of the truth of motherhood why are we not being told by those who guide our preparation for parenthood? We're warned about the baby blues. Why not the baby reds? GP and psychologist Dr Cathy Andronis, who is also the Royal Australian College of General Practitioners chair of psychological medicine, says it has to do with the bubble wrap society wants to put around expecting women. 'When women are pregnant we don't want to hurt them. We want them to be optimistic. But it gets extended to the point where people don't want to talk about [anger in motherhood], so there's a conspiracy of silence.' GPs are often the first port of call for concerns in the postpartum period, but plenty of new mums have told me they've been dismissed when they tried to raise their anger with their doctor. We heard Eleni's story earlier, of being told by her GP that she was a good parent because she felt bad when she yelled. Another mum of two told me a young male GP asked her if she had a hobby after she confided she wasn't coping. (Apparently, taking up yoga or knitting would fix it.) When she tried an older female GP, she was told it was okay because she would 'grow' from the stressful experience. There was also the mum of twins who admitted to a nurse in a specialist sleep support unit that she was 'just so angry' but was not given any further opportunity for conversation or support.

In country New South Wales, mum of two Kylie raised the issue of her anger at her six-week postpartum check-up, but felt she wasn't taken seriously. 'My GP said that it looked like I had it all together and I was doing a great job,' the 27-year-old told me. A midwife conducting a home visit didn't give her the standard mental health screening questionnaire because she thought she was 'doing just great. I feel like I still try very hard to project the image of a perfect mother even though inside I know I'm failing.' Kylie tells me she would like to speak to a psychologist, and wonders if she might benefit from antidepressant medication, but her experience with the GP has discouraged her from seeking further help.

Perth mum Jing, who had told me about the guilt she felt at bedtime, didn't see her particular struggles reflected anywhere, so she didn't feel they were worthy of support. 'I just felt like I was the only one in the world who couldn't handle motherhood and yelled at my kids all the time,' the

43-year-old stay-at-home mum said. 'You only hear about anxiety and depression, and I wasn't feeling those so I didn't seek out help. And the surveys they have mums do to try to pick up on depression don't ask the right questions.'

The COPE Australian Clinical Practice Guideline recommends that women are screened twice for signs of depression or anxiety while pregnant and twice again in the weeks and months after giving birth (although we know this doesn't always happen and some women are not screened at all). The most commonly used tool is the Edinburgh Postnatal Depression Scale (EPDS), which asks ten questions about how a new mum has felt over the past week. They touch on whether she has been sad, tearful, panicky, anxious, had difficulty sleeping or felt like harming herself. But none of the questions explicitly mention feeling frustrated, irritated, angry or out of control. The closest they come is a question that asks if the mum feels like 'things have been getting on top of me'.

A score of 13 or more on the EPDS can be a red flag for symptoms of depression or anxiety, and experts recommend that those women are referred for further assessment and support. However, a woman with a lower score could still be at risk if her answers have been affected by misunderstanding the questions or because of a fear of stigma or child removal. Many women have confided that they flat-out lied, giving the answers they knew the doctors or nurses wanted to hear. COPE has developed a digital version, iCOPE, which is helping to screen more women in 26 languages. Funded by the federal government, it has been used so far in Victoria, South Australia, Queensland, Tasmania and the Northern

Territory. COPE founder and executive director Dr Nicole Highet told me there is still stigma around raising perinatal mental health challenges because women often feel like they are failing in their role as a parent. Some women are 'very concerned about disclosing that they're not coping for fear of their child being removed', she said. However, early evidence indicates that being able to complete the iCOPE questions on a personal mobile phone is leading to higher rates of disclosure than being asked the question in person, usually by a GP, midwife or obstetrician.

Melbourne-based Dr Andronis told me that health professionals can be 'pulled into the same cautious approach that everyone has' about not wanting to say the A-word. 'Anger is a loaded term,' she said. 'Some women, they've almost put an armour around the word "anger" and they don't use it. So if you ask them "Are you angry?" they will say no because angry means that you're going to hurt someone.' Instead GPs may be inclined to 'use softer language' to approach the topic: 'They will use "irritable" – it's a gentler term to encompass anger.' There also may be a reluctance to open up such a large and nebulous topic given the average Medicare-subsidised GP visit can last as little as six minutes. 'Today's general practice prioritises quick medicine, people coming in with coughs and colds ... [to] see as many people as possible,' Dr Andronis said. 'So as soon as anger comes up [a GP may think], "Well, this is going to open up a Pandora's box."'

Part of the solution is to give GPs 'more reward' (read: better Medicare rebates) for spending longer with patients to have more complicated conversations. Higher rebates were promised at the 2025 federal election – but only for bulk-billed appointments, where the GP does not charge the patient anything above the government rebate. However, the rate of bulk-billing has been declining as the cost of running a medical business has risen.

Dr Andronis said it also helps to have a consistent connection with the same doctor. It can be incredibly difficult these days, with demand for GPs far outstripping supply, but she encourages us to look around for a doctor we can relate to. Doctors are 'not offended when a patient goes to someone else because they're a better fit', she assured me.

Our son was about 18 months old when I first realised I might need to talk to a professional about how I was feeling. I'd taken some annual leave from my paid job and, with a little extra headspace, it became clear that I wasn't being honest with myself, or anyone else, about how much noise there was in my head. That first appointment with the GP, on a warm Friday afternoon, was awkward. I didn't know where to start. It was hard to admit my outbursts, out loud and to a stranger who had a legal obligation to report if she thought a child was at risk. But she didn't judge or doubt me. She took me at my word, asked me what I wanted to do and gave me options. I still cringe when I think about how I struggled to articulate myself that day, but I cannot imagine how the shame would have been magnified if I had been dismissed.

A way to manage

As we go through the rest of this book, I'll break down in more detail some of the factors that can spark anger in motherhood, from biological and psychological to social and structural. Everything from PMS to patriarchy can trigger mum rage. Initially I felt most of my triggers were physiological, chief among them lack of sleep. So I wanted to better understand how anger manifests in my brain, why it is harder to control when I'm tired or hungry, which hormones are at play and when. But I also knew that these were only the yellow and orange flames of my mum rage, the ones flickering up and down around the sides of a big pot holding all the ingredients in my motherhood soup. Fuelling the fire below were the burning embers of unfairness, overwhelm, monotony, uncertainty, loss of freedom and identity. These took a lot longer to register, obscured by the bright flames, and they are much harder to confront. I won't ever fully douse them, but with the right amount of attention my motherhood soup can remain at a gentle simmer, without boiling over.

The problem was that when I first went looking for ways to manage my mum rage, I found that anger usually featured as a side dish, rather than being the main meal. Books, films and podcasts on the reality of motherhood are more common now but, still, few put fury front and centre. Much of what I found early on either ignored it, trivialised it, made me feel worse about it or gave me (frankly) useless advice. I didn't want a step-by-step workbook for which I had no time or patience. I didn't need a dense history of feminist theory to understand that I was pissed off about the inequality inherent in parenting (particularly in heterosexual couples). I was overwhelmed by the conflicting advice of parenting experts and was in no state to take on their lessons. I needed to know what was going on inside my body, but all I could find were basic public health websites or impenetrable medical articles I was too tired to make sense of (until I had to for this book). Like those in the Angry Mums Club, what I really wanted was to know that I wasn't alone. And then I wanted to know what had worked for anyone who had managed to turn down the heat beneath their own bubbling pot.

What follows is not a self-help guide or a parenting manual. But it has become, for me, a way to manage. Once you understand the drivers of your own mum rage, you may realise that you need to do some much deeper work, perhaps with the help of a professional. This book is not about how to do that work, but it may help you get to a place where you have the time and energy to do it, if you need.

Awareness

The first step for me was awareness. I didn't know mum rage was a thing until I experienced it. Safe to say I'm 'aware' now – and if you're reading this book you are too. If nothing else, I hope this book raises more awareness – especially among those expecting their first child – that anger in motherhood is common, not shameful. (Perhaps consider gifting a copy at the next baby shower you attend, rather than a onesie the kid might never wear.)

Analysis

Once I became aware, I'll be honest, I just marinated in that for a while. *Gee, I'm angry, everything is making me angry, everything is hard*, and so on. But eventually I had to move on to analysis. I know this sounds like it's going to use a lot of brain power that none of us has to spare, but it doesn't have to be deep, meditative reflection or a series of spreadsheets. At first I was just looking at the low-hanging fruit. *Am I tired? Am I hungry? Am I sore? Am I fed up with staying at home with a baby who does a poo in the bath while my partner goes out for dinner?* Some things will be a quick fix: go to bed early, eat a muesli bar, take some paracetamol. Others will require more time and work. You know, like negotiating better gender equality in your household or pay packet. But we can get to those later, after you're feeling more rested. You can't smash the patriarchy when you're sleep deprived and hangry.

Asking for help

The next step for me was to start removing some of the irritants and obstacles I'd identified in order to make space – physically and mentally – to tackle the bigger stuff. I needed more sleep, to move my body, to have some time to myself.

To get this I had to ask for some help, largely in the form of babysitting. Chances are whatever is on your list is going to be at least somewhat eased by calling in reinforcements. The key is to ask early – before you start feeling so burned out and cranky that you don't want to interact with anyone else and just resign yourself to soldiering on in autopilot. The sooner you ask for help, the sooner you'll figure out who's willing to give it. I'd love to say that offers just come flying at you once you have a child. Sometimes they do – from special people who've been there, survived it and have the time to give back. And I've been lucky to have those people in my life. But if you're having kids at the same time as all your friends or siblings, they're probably also too exhausted and busy to offer much assistance, so you're going to have to figure out who in your orbit has the capacity and inclination, and just straight-out ask. I really struggled with this at first, but always felt better once I did.

Automating

Eventually, I realised that the more I could automate the help, the less I had to think or worry about it. Automating allows you to ask once and then have the situation repeat without having to ask again. For example, I asked our children's grandparents to look after them initially for an hour or two here and there. But this added to my mental load, thinking about when and how to ask them, if it was too often or inconvenient. After a while we settled on roughly the same time on the same day each week. This system changes if someone is sick, busy or goes on holidays (them, not us!), but for the most part it is now a set-and-forget situation. You could also have your groceries delivered on the same day each week or rotate the same old seven meals for dinner.

Another way to think about automating is to ask yourself what you can outsource, or even stop altogether. This can be a really difficult question to answer for the majority of us who have internalised the demands of 'intensive mothering', a term coined by sociologist Sharon Hays in the 1990s and one that you'll become more acquainted with later in this book. In short, this dominant understanding of mothering has us believing that mums should be the primary carer for our precious children, who deserve every opportunity in life and every moment of our attention. But if you're willing to shush your inner critic (and you must!), automating could be deciding that you don't have to bake all the kids' birthday cakes from scratch (you can buy one from the shop) and that they can do some of the household chores themselves. It could also be setting up a speaker in their rooms to play a bedtime story on the nights when you can't read one more page or, if you can afford it, biting the bullet and buying that robo-vacuum to patrol the crumb-covered floors on your behalf.

Actively resisting

Be warned: by this point, you'll be making some changes that might catch a few people off guard. It might result in some pushback – from your partner, your extended family, your boss or even your kids. And your inner critic may be the loudest protester. But if you want anything to change, you'll need to summon the energy to actively resist all that. Everything we've talked about up to now has been about giving you back time and energy so you can use it to fight the important fights. A crucial part of this step is knowing what is worth fighting for and what to let go. Some things actually don't need to be resisted. Why can't your kid wear that ridiculous outfit in public? Is it really so bad if they eat cereal or popcorn for dinner some nights?

But in other cases it is vital to resist, and you're going to have to get comfortable saying no. No to requests to do more, make more, organise more, solve more. The problem is that other people benefit when you go above and beyond, and your decision to resist their expectations (or the expectations you set with your previous behaviour) can spark backlash. But, in dual-parent households, why should it always be you who changes the pooey nappy? Why should it always be you who picks the kids up from childcare? Single parents might not have someone to tag out with but there is no need to make things harder by trying to keep up with everyone else. Just because other kids do three extra-curricular activities a week, or take homemade sushi for lunch, doesn't mean your kid has to. It's going to feel weird and awkward at first, and it will take a while to see change, but you must protect your reclaimed time and space.

Alone time

This is the big one, the thing most worth fighting for. To get time alone I have to actively resist both my inner critic and my default reluctance to ask someone else to look after my kids 'just' so I can do something for myself. Absurdly, this hesitation is almost strongest when I'm asking my partner. Perhaps it's because he is also the parent of these little cherubs who deprive us of sleep and social lives, and he's desperate for a break as well. But it is my strong belief that time to ourselves, without the relentless responsibilities of child-rearing, is essential to sustainable parenting. I'm not talking about a two-week trip to Tahiti, but I do mean more than five minutes alone in the loo. Without decent respite it is extremely difficult to short-circuit the build-up of triggers before the mum rage pot boils over.

Axing the guilt

When you finally get that time alone, you've got to axe the guilt about it. None of the rest of it matters much if you are consumed by guilt, anxiety and overthinking every time you get a moment to yourself. It took me a while to stop clock-watching on solo outings, or repeatedly checking in on the kids whenever they were being looked after by someone else. Guilt can be an important signal that we've gone against our values in parenting – for instance, if we smack our child when this is something we don't want to do. But guilt is a strong contributor to mum rage because it also, often falsely, signals to us that we have failed in some way as a mother. Even if that is a failure to live up to an unreasonable or unrealistic standard. Our default response can be to get defensive or to try even harder, but that will just lead to burnout. So when you get that support and that time, do *not* waste it feeling guilty.

There you have it – awareness, analysis, asking for help, automating what you can, actively resisting the expectations or the pushback, getting some alone time and axing the guilt about it – that's how I've grappled with my mum rage. It's still a work in progress, but it has made a huge difference. Over the course of this book, we'll examine some of the most common triggers and how these approaches can help avoid or lessen them. The first step is awareness. So what even is anger?

What is anger?

'It comes out of nowhere.'

That's how so many mums describe it when the fury erupts. It seems to just burst out, taking them by surprise. Some can sense it building, over hours or days, but feel powerless to stop it. Others describe a constant, low-level irritation, a foul mood that flares.

Put very, very simply, anger is an emotion, triggered by something, that usually prompts us to take some sort of action. Despite being a common emotion, anger gets a bad rap. People are still really reluctant to name the feeling and we often reach for a watered-down version, like 'irritated' or 'frustrated'. Anger is not sympathetic. If we're crying because we're sad or overwhelmed, our tears might elicit empathy and support, but anger tends to provoke judgement or push people away, which can leave us even more isolated. And anger is definitely not seen as a feminine emotion. Indeed, Australian Association of Psychologists member Annabel Hales says women she sees are 'more comfortable presenting with depression or anxiety. That's far more palatable. But to be angry or to display rage or fury … no.' However, Hales regards anger as a useful emotion. 'It provides clarity, lets us check in with our value systems, if our boundaries are being crossed, and it precipitates action,' she says.

The problem is sometimes (or in fact oftentimes) in motherhood, we can't address the trigger by doing something. If you're angry because a baby won't stop crying and you've tried feeding, changing, cuddling and rocking that baby then you hit a brick wall in terms of what you can do. As Adelaide psychologist Jo Hamilton put it when we spoke at her suburban office, 'you've done everything, there is no action you can take,' but you still have the physical reaction to being unable to comfort your baby, unable to make the distressing crying noise stop. 'That physiological response, the cascade of cortisol and adrenaline, it's got nowhere to go, so then it could come out as rage,' Hamilton said.

An outburst can bring some relief (even if short-lived). As parenting expert, author and mum-of-three Lael Stone told the *Mum Mind Unpacked* podcast: 'The body wants to move its anger ... [It] needs to push against something, it needs to shake, it needs to yell, it needs to rip up things, it needs to snap things.' As Stone spoke I was reminded of that viral TikTok video of a mother hurling ice cubes into her bathtub. And my relative who used to raise her arms and yell up at the ceiling, rather than at her children, to shift her frustrated energy about the toys scattered all over the floor. On the podcast, Stone revealed that mum rage 'is probably one of the biggest topics I talk about with women'. She too felt, when her children were little, 'this anger and rage that ... I was shocked by'. It comes from needing a break, Stone said, but also from taking on too much, not being able to say no and trying to keep a lid on a 'backlog' of feelings and frustrations that we haven't been able – or taught – to express. 'It feels almost safer to get angry at everyone around us ... than to actually pause and go, "What is here for me? What am I avoiding feeling?"'[1]

Like Stone, most of the psychologists and sociologists I spoke to for this book stressed that, in the context of motherhood, anger is an emotion usually triggered by an unmet need. It might feel like it's the toddler refusing to put on their shoes, the spilt breastmilk you spent half an hour pumping, or the teenager's rude retort that you're responding to, but really it's your need to be listened to, your need for things to go to plan, or your need for respect. The experts also told me anger is usually trying to tell us something is wrong, that we are facing an injustice or a threat, and this warning system is not necessarily a bad thing. As sociologist Dr Sophie Brock says, in many cases an angry mother is reacting 'in a very rational and logical way to the circumstances that she's been put in'. Ain't that the truth.

So it might feel as if a burst of anger comes out of nowhere but there is always a trigger, or series of triggers. And there is usually a build-up, even if we don't see it coming. Here, awareness and analysis come into play. How can we identify our triggers and recognise when they are mounting? Members of the Angry Mums Club said that during an outburst they felt physical sensations like tingling, buzzing, tense muscles, racing heart, headache, nausea or a surge of energy. These feelings persisted for many of them after the blow-up. The most common after-effects were feeling drained or tired (52 per cent), having a racing mind (44 per cent) and still feeling agitated (37 per cent).

What is going on in our body and our brain when we experience this? Why does it feel like our emotions take over before our rational brain has any say in it? I'm no scientist (I'm not even a science journalist) but I'm going to do my best to bring together all the reading and interviews I've done to explain the neuroscience of anger to busy, tired mums who find it hard to concentrate at the best of times. Here goes ...

First, we need to meet a few key players. You might have heard of the *amygdalae*, two little almond-shaped parts of your brain that are responsible for monitoring threats and generating emotions. They sit at the base of your brain and are one of its oldest and most primitive parts. The job of the amygdalae has long been to keep us alive by reacting quickly and decisively to incoming information, particularly threats.

Near to the amygdalae are the *hypothalamus, thalamus* and *hippocampus*. These are part of what is known as the *limbic system*, the middle part of our brain concerned largely with emotions and memory. The hypothalamus is occupied mostly with involuntary processes like our heart rate, breathing, digestion and hormone regulation. The thalamus is particularly responsible for taking in and relaying information to the correct part of the brain. And the hippocampus helps us put things in perspective and send our important memories to long-term storage.

In the same neighbourhood of the brain is the *pituitary gland*. Together with the hypothalamus, it forms part of a crucial pathway responsible for our emotional reactions, particularly to stress, known as the *HPA axis* – H for hypothalamus, P for pituitary gland, and A for *adrenal glands*. These two triangle-shaped glands are actually not in your

What is anger?

brain, but down on your kidneys. They secrete hormones, including cortisol and adrenaline, which prompt us to act and which contribute to the hot flushes, surges of energy or dizziness we might feel when our emotions are heightened.

The final pieces of the puzzle are in the *cortex*. This is the outermost part of our brain and the newest, evolutionarily speaking. It's our common-sense brain region and the part responsible for helping us do things like regulate, re-evaluate, rationalise and strategise. Different parts of this outer band of brain (we'll call them cortices, collectively) specialise in different things: vision, hearing, movement, speech, etc. Of particular relevance to us is the *prefrontal cortex*, which sits right behind our foreheads and is where the real higher order thinking and decision-making happens. And the *orbital frontal cortex*, directly above our eye sockets, which helps us weigh up decisions and (importantly for anger in motherhood) can override our emotional impulses. But 'can' is the crucial word. When those emotional little amygdalae get too excited, they can sideline the prefrontal and orbital frontal cortices. This is often referred to as 'emotional hijacking'.[2]

Every moment of every day our brain is taking in information, deciding what to ignore, how to respond, what to remember. Very simply speaking, there are two pathways the brain can use to do this: the quick, emotional way or the slower, more rational way.

The first, fast pathway goes something like this:

1) Our senses pick up some information. Let's go with the example of our eyes registering a dark, thin shape on the front doorstep as we're rushing out to work.

2) Our thalamus, whose job it is to pick up and relay information, takes in this image from our visual cortices and sends it out for a brief assessment in the memory centres of our brain.
3) The message comes back quickly that the shape is a snake.
4) The thalamus sends that info straight over to the amygdalae, who rifle through their memory cards (which have a heavily weighted 'fear' deck) and see that snakes are associated with danger and pose a likely threat.
5) The amygdalae make the snap decision that we need to take action to protect ourselves, so they send a signal to our adrenal glands to pump out some cortisol quick smart. This gives us the extra push we need to shoot out our hand and slam the door shut.

Now let's rewind and take the slower route:

1) Our eyes register the dark, thin shape on the doorstep.
2) Our thalamus takes in that information from the visual cortices and sends it out for a bit more examination.
3) This time our hippocampus, whose job it is to help put things in perspective, gets the memo and starts riffling through its back catalogue, trying to find a match. It sees something similar – a snake – but it's not an exact match. There also aren't a

What is anger?

lot of snakes in the memory bank. There are lots of sticks, though – also dark and thin, and much more likely to have ended up on our suburban doorstep.

4) In the moment it has taken for the hippocampus to do this, our amygdalae might have jumped in first with a signal to the adrenal glands for a quick squirt of cortisol, giving us a start. But hippocampus swiftly follows up with a 'stop' signal, telling the adrenal glands to stand down.

5) Our orbital frontal cortex (the bit that can override our emotions) is now able to step in and temper our reaction. Our prefrontal cortex (our thinking brain) can direct us to reach down, pick up the stick and chuck it onto the front lawn so we don't trip over it (a possible future threat).

Now let's apply this process to that moment I shared, at the start of this book, when I flew into a rage after being woken by my partner going to bed:

1) Lying in the spare room, my ears pick up the sound of the handle clicking into place as he closes our bedroom door.
2) My thalamus, whose job it is to pick up and relay information, takes in the unexpected sound from my auditory cortices, coupled with the fact that my visual cortices are telling me it's pitch dark. That information is going straight to the amygdalae.

3) They riffle through their memory cards and see that noises that wake me up could signal danger, and not getting enough sleep is a potential threat to me and my ability to take care of a very dependent baby.
4) The amygdalae decide that the best course of action, in the short amount of time I have to consider all this, is to shout down to the adrenal glands to 'deploy the cortisol'. This will help launch me out of bed and confront the source of the potential threat. Before the hippocampus can even start flicking through its albums, my amygdalae and I are off and running.

Rewinding, let's see what could have happened if my brain took the slower route that night:

1) Lying in bed, my ears pick up the sound of the bedroom door handle clicking into place as my partner goes to bed.
2) My thalamus, whose job it is to pick up and relay information, takes in the sound from my auditory cortices, and the pitch-black info from the visual cortices. Unsure exactly where I am or what's going on, the thalamus decides to send the info elsewhere for further investigation.
3) My hippocampus takes the call and starts riffling through its memory cards. It recognises the click sound as coming from the bedroom door (a sound tucked into my long-term memory bank after

What is anger?

hearing it many times before) and assesses that the noise is short-lived and unlikely to present an ongoing impediment to falling asleep.
4) The amygdalae were all ready to fire up the adrenal glands but hippocampus jumps in to tell them there is no major threat to my sleep or my ability to care for the baby.
5) Hippocampus sends out the signal for the adrenal glands to cease fire and we all take a deep breath and roll over.

The complexity of this process, and the mystery, is that the same thing can sometimes trigger an angry rush and other times not. In terms of human evolution, the slower pathway is a more recent development. It uses parts of the brain that evolved much later to allow for further examination of context. The first pathway is a well-worn route designed to keep us safe, to be quick but not necessarily accurate. Jo Hamilton, also a member of the Australian Association of Psychologists, says this is because we evolved to overreact, rather than underreact. She gives an example from evolution, of an early human spotting a suspect shape in the distance: if they think, 'Oh, that's probably not a lion,' but it turns out to be one, then they might be killed. But if they take off running and it turns out to be a cat, well, better safe than sorry.

It's still not entirely clear why it goes one way or another, but the space between the trigger and our response is crucial. A lot of the time, rational human brains can use that space (however minimal) to make a helpful decision. But when other factors like sleep deprivation, hunger, pain, fear or overwhelming emotions are part of the mix, our thinking brain can't stick its nose in fast enough. There's no reasoning your way out of an emotional response and you can feel like you've lost your mind. 'With fury and rage, you're literally hijacked by the experience,' Perth-based clinical and counselling psychologist Annabel Hales explained to me. 'There's a powerlessness to rage. It takes over. That incredibly primal rage feeling is very different to anger.' This has come as a shock to many of the mums Hales has worked with over more than 23 years, who say that depth of feeling is 'uncharacteristic'. However, it shouldn't really be surprising, given we have evolved to have fight or flight reactions. 'That feeling is in our body, and it's still there, it's in our wiring, it hasn't gone anywhere,' Hales said. 'Now we're not fighting the sabre-toothed tiger … but it's still coming up to the surface in different ways.'

Fear is often an undercurrent to anger. I mentioned earlier how I've been set off by panic over a sick child refusing to take medicine. I've heard a version of this story from countless other mums. We're not really angry at the kid. We're worried about them. It's the same for the mum who told me she berated her tweenage son because he never looked properly before stepping out onto a road, as well as those of us who mothered through the peak of the COVID-19 pandemic, when everything felt like a threat and our collective nerves were frayed. Among the Angry Mums Club, almost one in five said fear or panic about the safety of a child was a trigger for an outburst. And fear of failure counts too. Pre-pandemic surveys of European mothers found their fears of failing their children, or failing to live up to expectations, became

What is anger?

'overwhelming'.³ First-time parents in the United Kingdom spoke of the anxiety induced by the 'absolute fear' of what the night would bring and 'fear of [the baby's] crying, fear of not knowing what to do'.⁴

We might not like to think of them this way, but our children also pose threats to us all the time. They threaten our sleep, our peace, our ability to eat regular meals (which can be interpreted by our ancient internal systems as a threat to our survival). They can even – unintentionally, of course – pose a physical threat. When I spoke to Hales, she recounted an example from when she worked as a nanny, before having a child of her own. She was changing a baby's nappy and the baby kicked her. 'It really hurt and my first reaction was to push back,' she said (adding that her thinking brain was able to intervene in that case).

But what if, instead of a young nanny caring for someone else's baby, it was a sleep-deprived mum who was also responsible for a preschooler and a pre-teen? She might have been woken early and realised there was no milk in the fridge to make a much-needed coffee. She's parenting solo while her FIFO partner is away for work, so she has to get all three kids dressed and off to their respective childcare, kindergarten and school on time before she lands at her part-time job. And when the baby on the change table kicks her – two minutes before she needs to leave – his foot is covered in zinc cream that smears all over her only clean, black uniform. Boom. She melts down.

This mum's morning is a classic example of what researcher Dolf Zillmann calls a 'sequence of provocations'. I first came across this University of Alabama professor of communication and psychology when I read Minna Dubin's *New York Times* essay on mother rage. Dubin explained Zillmann's theory about how anger builds on itself so that 'by the third or fourth rage trigger, the person is reacting on a level 10 in response to a misplaced key or a dropped spoon'.[5] I thought, *Yes, exactly!* And I wanted to know more. Zillmann's original explanation of this process appears in a chapter he wrote in a scientific handbook titled 'Mental control of angry aggression'. In it, he addresses how the 'sequence of provocations' triggers our nervous system. As each new trigger comes, it 'rides the tails' of the one before. This means that we can remain in a heightened state of irritation and vigilance 'for hours and days' after the initial trigger.[6]

In the notes section of my phone, I recorded one such sequence in our house. I had been unwell for a few days prior and was parenting solo that day. I took the kids to a playground and they both fell asleep in the pram on the walk home (which was part of the plan), but when we got inside, one kid woke up suddenly and started crying, which woke up the other kid, who then wouldn't transfer to bed for their usual nap (not part of the plan). The rest of the afternoon was a battle. At some point, one of the kids was ripping leaves off our blueberry bush while the other was jumping on the couch. Finally, it was bedtime. I'd read three stories and was trying to make my exit from one of the children's bedrooms. They kept popping up and asking for more food, even though they'd had two dinners, and I finally snapped. 'ENOUGH!' I roared. 'BE QUIET AND GO TO SLEEP!' And I stalked out. For the entire day, one trigger had been riding the tails of the one before it and I couldn't hold it in any longer.

What is anger?

Zillmann explains how the nervous system is involved in this cascade in two different ways. To grasp what he's on about, we need to understand a key fact about our adrenal glands (which, we know from earlier in this chapter, sit on top of our kidneys). They have two parts that release different hormones. Very simply, the *medulla* is the inside bit and the *cortex* is the outside bit. Zillman tells us that the *adrenomedullary system* (the inner part of our adrenal glands) responds to acute triggers (say, stepping on LEGO blocks that weren't packed away) by releasing hormones to provide a quick burst of energy for one action (perhaps swearing as we kick aside the remaining errant LEGO blocks). In contrast, the *adrenocortical system* (the outer part of the adrenal glands) responds to ongoing stressors (say, a constant state of mess around the house) and releases steroid hormones for energy over an extended period of time.

I think of this second system as our baseline level of agitation and the first system as our spike level. The two systems affect each other. Heightened activity in your baseline (from a constantly messy house) puts you in a state of vigilance, so when you step on that piece of LEGO the anger spikes higher than it might otherwise. People who are already stressed by everyday life will, Zillmann says, bring that into a new conflict (say, with the child who left out the LEGO) and this makes it much more likely that we're going to blow up about the acute trigger.

If there are enough triggers in the sequence and not enough time between them for the nervous system to reset, it makes emotional hijacking more likely. As Zillmann explains, the part of our brain that can override the impulse to lash out under ordinary levels of nervous system agitation 'fails to operate' at extreme levels.[7] We're just too far gone. Even the understanding of likely consequences (like the neighbours hearing us swear when we kick aside the LEGO) is not enough to halt the aggression. (Been there ...)

When we're at that extreme level, Zillmann says we are more likely to fall back on habits or 'well-rehearsed reactions' in the absence of our better judgement.[8] This was alarming to read as it reinforced my fear that the more I yell, the more I will yell. Thinking back to how our brain can take the fast or slow road to make a decision, the difficulty seems to be that once we form habits, they tend to be the fast road. If we develop a habit of overreacting and yelling then that becomes like 'a super freeway' in our brain, as psychologist Jo Hamilton (a mum of two grown-up kids) put it. And when we're trying to change our response, to form a new habit of engaging the thinking brain (like pausing instead of yelling), that is much harder. It's more like taking 'a little path in a wheat field, riddled with spiders and farmers shouting at you', Hamilton suggested. With this in mind, the best way to change is gently. 'If you shout at yourself and beat up on yourself, your brain just shuts down even more,' she said.

Clinical psychologist Dr Nicole Williams, also a mum of two in Adelaide, challenges us to think about an *experience* of anger, rather than an *issue* or *problem* with it. 'A lot of the work I do is helping women not to buy into the stigma about it ... to understand that it is a normal human emotion,' she told me. 'It will often blow their mind a little bit because their experience has been that anger is really scary and dangerous.' If they don't want any part of it, then it's to be expected that they'll become self-critical and then feel guilty – and 'then we get into that horrible cycle'. Dr Williams acknowledges there are kinds of anger that are not safe but points out it is the behaviour that can be a problem, rather than the emotion. 'It's okay to feel the thing,' she reminds us. The important bit is what you do with it.

What about the dads?

If that's how mums' brains and nervous systems work, it's the same for dads, right? They get angry too. Of course they do. So why aren't I writing a book about dad rage? At least one in ten dads experience mental health challenges around parenthood. They too feel pressured and overwhelmed and grieve their old lives. I've spoken to fathers for this book who have felt the same frustration and anger I have, especially if they have taken on the role of primary carer in their family. I've come to believe that there is a direct link between the amount of time we spend with our children – rather than our gender or what our kids call us – and the likelihood of experiencing anger in parenthood. More time spent caring for the kids is more time we have to answer questions, separate squabbling siblings, add items to the mental load, avert disasters … you get the picture. Sure, that could be any of us spending a lot of time with our kids, but the reality, in Australia and many other countries, is that it is more often mums who spend more hours a day, more days a week, in the role of primary carer. So this book is about the everyday irritations, stresses and structural barriers that leave those mums silently fuming, or screaming their heads off. We'll learn more in later chapters about how much of the mum rage out there is directed at dads (or any partners, ex-partners or co-parents) because mums feel they are shouldering too much of the burden of parenting. Many don't understand how they ended up as the default parent and they can't see a way back to a more equal footing.

The dominant gender stereotypes we've grown up with in Australia mean that we also have different expectations about how men and women will respond to frustration. When a bloke rages (but, to be clear, not to the level of abuse), we are more likely to think he is putting his foot down, drawing a line, winning. It's dad coming in to sort things out. As we've already heard from psychologists, girls and women are not encouraged to express themselves in the same way, so when we do, we are going against the socialisation that descends on us from birth. Angry women are still seen (unfairly) as shrill, hysterical, overreacting. It's mum 'not coping'.

Men and women also appear to think differently about the transition to parenthood and how it changes them. A 1985 assessment by American researchers, while done some years ago, remains relevant. Men and women in relationships, who had become parents, were asked to fill in a pie chart to show how much of their lives they attributed to different identities: parent, worker and partner. Mum's *worker* piece of pie was pretty skinny while her *parent* slice widened to almost 40 per cent of her identity. In contrast, dad threw himself further into the role of worker and felt only 20 per cent of his identity was tied to parenting.[1] (We'll look later at the cultural and structural factors that contribute to this.)

There are about four million families with children living in Australia. The 2021 Australian Bureau of Statistics (ABS) Census recorded about 2.9 million two-parent households and another million-plus single-parent homes (80 per cent of which were single-mother households).[2] There were almost 24,000 families where the adults were in a same-sex marriage. Other data from 2021 shows the dad chose to stay home and be the primary carer in only 2.5 per cent of couples with a child under one year of age at that time.[3]

Since 2010, eligible Australians starting, or growing, a family have been able to apply for paid parental leave for the primary carer. Almost everyone who has taken up this option has been female. Australian Institute of Family Studies (AIFS) analysis shows 94.3 per cent of the almost 1.8 million people who received the payment up to the end of 2022 were women with a male partner. The next largest group of recipients was about 90,000 single mums. More than 9400 men, with a female partner, elected to receive the payment, but they weren't necessarily the primary carer because about 70 per cent shared it with their partner. The remaining payments went to 8800 women with a female partner, 440-odd men with a male partner and 220-odd single men.[4]

Paid parental leave is offered when a baby enters the family. But what's happening by the time that baby is ready for school? A study by AIFS researcher Jennifer Baxter looked at who four- and five-year-old children spent their time with. She found they were 'at all times more likely to be with their mother than their father'.[5] At. All. Times. Baxter was working with data from 2010, but everything I've heard and read while writing this book suggests not a whole lot has changed in many Australian households.

It's a similar story when we look at parents' employment patterns. Back in 1991, 32 per cent of Australian families had a stay-at-home mum. That figure dropped to one-quarter by 2016 as more women entered or rejoined the workforce. However, the proportion of dads staying home with the kids hasn't budged from 3 or 4 per cent.[6] Other ABS data from 2023–24 shows women are more likely to miss out on job opportunities because they are shouldering the majority of the child-care load. Among women who wanted to take up a job or more hours but couldn't, 45 per cent said the main barrier was child-caring responsibilities. That was almost six times the proportion of men held back from entering the labour market because they had to look after their kids.[7] And at home the division of unpaid labour is still seriously skewed. In 2019, Aussie mothers living with a partner were doing almost 21 hours more unpaid work, like cleaning, cooking and child care, each week than fathers.[8]

On these numbers, it seems clear that Australian mums are far more likely than anyone else in their household to be buffeted by the relentless provocations of parenting. We'll get into more detail about what drives a lot of this and sets mum up as the 'default parent' but, for now, let these figures be your answer to the 'What about the dads?' question.

And to the dads who *do* spend more hours with their children than their parenting partner does, who change more nappies, wake up more often overnight, make more school lunches and cover more kilometres dropping teens to weekend sport or part-time jobs, may you feel seen within these pages too. Because, while this is a book by a mum for mums, it is really for anyone who has spent long enough with a child to reach their breaking point ... and then had to do it again and again until bedtime, and then all over again the next day and the next.

What if you're not the 'real' mum?

There are about 287,000 births recorded around Australia each year,[1] but mums aren't just made in the delivery room. Leanne's four children were all birthed by other women. To her kids she is 'Mum', but in so many situations she is made to feel like she's 'not the real mum'. The sting of that judgement is worsened by the fact that Leanne and her husband endured repeated miscarriages. 'I don't know everybody's story but it just felt so easy for everybody else,' she told me. 'Especially in my early 30s when everybody was dropping babies all over the place. I got angry but I had to internalise it because you have to be really happy for everybody.' Being, as Leanne puts it, 'excluded from the mum club' is paradoxically one of her biggest mum rage triggers. 'No one knows what to say to you. I had a lot of friends who just stopped talking to me because it was easier. I would have to remove myself from another situation – here's another place I can't go or another thing I'm going to get excluded from – just to try and protect my heart.'

She's not alone. Many women and men told researchers at COPE about the pain and resentment of watching others fall pregnant. Some reported 'strong feelings of anger or jealousy'. COPE's research for its The Truth awareness campaign found the perception that pregnancy 'should be a happy time', and a lack of understanding about the challenges pregnancy and parenthood could bring, meant people did not feel able to speak honestly about how they felt.[2]

Leanne said her grief and anger were compounded by feeling excluded. 'I was working that hard and I wasn't recognised as their mum ... all while I'm losing babies. I was doing so much mothering and then people would be like, "What's their real mum doing?" It made me angry, and embarrassed.' In fact, it made Leanne furious but she 'stuffed it down', until the feelings made their way to the surface. 'Frustrations came out because it was like, "Why am I bothering if nobody is recognising anything I'm doing?" I was doing all of that but not given that title of "Mum".'

This feeling of being taken for granted is a common trigger for anger in motherhood, whether it's our children taking for granted that we'll pick up after them, our partner taking for granted that we'll cook dinner, or our boss taking for granted that we'll meet the deadline regardless of what's going on at home. It is even more painful for women who are told they are 'just' a stepmum, foster mum, carer or adoptive mother. 'I would walk through fire for these kids, and people take that away from me on the daily,' Leanne said. 'There's no explaining that rage of somebody taking that power from me. I'm powerless over my fertility. I'm powerless over the kids because I'm not their biological parent. Everybody makes decisions on their behalf, but they would never question an actual birth mother. That's a special kind of anger, that one.'

If biological mothers feel stigma, judgement or fear about admitting mum rage, the risk is even higher for those who become parents through fostering, adoption, kinship or blended families. 'The rules are so different,' said Leanne, whose family is one of about 24,200 across Australia to have at least one child in state care placed with them.[3] 'You have to be really careful because anyone can make a report against you, even if they just don't like your tone.' Does the extra scrutiny stop mums like Leanne asking for help? 'Absolutely,' she replied without hesitation. 'I have to pretend everything is okay. I don't need a fucking medal, but every now and then just call me their mum. Or at least give me a break and don't judge me.'

Part Two

Triggered

It's my hormones, Doc

The baby blues hit me haaaaard a couple of days after I gave birth to our first child. My mum's warning that they would come had helped somewhat, but it was kind of like knowing a tsunami wave is rushing in to shore and looking around for a surfboard. I remember sitting in our room on the maternity ward, holding our newly arrived bundle, and not being able to stop the tears. I was awestruck, in love and incredibly grateful that our daughter was out safely. She was perfection in miniature, and I couldn't quite believe she was real. I was also overwhelmed and confused, and that was in the quieter moments. What was more characteristic of those first few days was high-pitched wailing (the baby, not me). We were having trouble figuring out breastfeeding, my milk hadn't come in and our tiny girl was starving. At one point, the midwives offered to take her for a few hours so I could get some sleep. I begrudgingly agreed and felt mildly panic-stricken the whole time (unable, then, to axe the guilt). Every newborn squawk from the corridor made me wonder if it was her – and then I felt worse for not being able to recognise my own child's cry (even though we'd only met properly the day before). I was a mess.

According to the Royal Women's Hospital in Melbourne, the baby blues can affect up to 80 per cent of people who give birth.[1] Exactly why some are affected and others aren't is unclear. Dr Oscar Serrallach, in his 2018 book *The Postnatal Depletion Cure*, describes the likely cause of the baby blues as a swift drop in progesterone, estrogen and cortisol, 'coupled with an immediate increase' in prolactin (the lactation hormone) and a resurgence in cortisol levels.[2] Whatever it was, when it happened to me, I felt anxious, sad and self-critical – but not yet rageful.

When women or girls get emotional, there is a strong tendency to blame it on hormones. How often have we heard or said, 'It's just that time of the month.' The influence of hormones is used, particularly by men, as a convenient way to dismiss or distract from other factors. I want to be clear that I am *not* pinning the entirety of mum rage on hormones here. There are *so* many reasons why mums are angry – enough to write a whole book about, in fact. Hormones are just one possible contributor. But let's not kid ourselves that they don't have any impact. Among the 200 members of the Angry Mums Club, half said hormone fluctuations or their menstrual cycle were contributing factors to their overall anger, and a third said they played a role in the moment of an outburst.

So-called 'sex hormones' – estrogen, progesterone and testosterone – probably spring to mind first, but hormones are a broad group of chemical messengers that play a role in many bodily functions. You might recognise the names of others like cortisol and adrenaline (the stressy ones) or melatonin (the sleepy one). Hormones are made all over the body, including in your brain, ovaries, gut and adrenal glands.

Professor Jayashri Kulkarni has spent most of her professional life focusing on the 'very real' impact of hormones on women's mental health. The Indian-Australian psychiatrist and mother of two adult daughters wrote her PhD in the late 1990s on women and psychosis. In 2019, she was awarded an Order of Australia (AM) for her contribution to medicine. Early in her career she worked in a large mental health hospital where the female patients were experiencing severe symptoms, including psychosis and auditory hallucinations. When she asked what brought these on, the women would repeatedly tell her, 'It's my hormones, Doc.' In some cases, after the women were prescribed the hormone estrogen, these distressing symptoms would vanish. This was when Professor Kulkarni realised how the significant impacts of sex hormones on the brain were being overlooked. In an interview on the ABC's *Conversations* she explained how, rather than diminishing women by attributing their difficulties to hormones, we should recognise that we are incredibly lucky to have hormonal treatments available that mean women aren't held back unnecessarily by debilitating but manageable conditions.[3]

A quick refresher for those who may not have thought too much about this since puberty or a years-ago pregnancy: a textbook menstrual cycle runs for 28 days. On day one your period starts. While you're bleeding, estrogen levels are low. They start to climb during the follicular phase, when your ovary is maturing an egg for release. Around day 14, at ovulation, the egg bursts out of the follicle. Estrogen levels peak at this point, before tapering off during the luteal phase of the cycle (that's the week or two leading up to your next period). Estrogen is at its lowest levels seven to ten days before you begin bleeding again. For women who are most sensitive to hormonal fluctuations, these are the danger days. This is when many will experience symptoms of premenstrual syndrome (better known as PMS) like bloating, breast tenderness and food cravings, as well as irritability or sadness.

From her office in Melbourne, Professor Kulkarni explained to me that estrogen has been shown to be 'protective' for our brain, meaning higher levels help with concentration, learning, memory and mood. This could be why managing all these things feels harder in the week or so before your period. There are receptors all throughout our brain to receive estrogen and the messages it brings, and they are particularly concentrated in the limbic system (the part of the brain we learned about earlier that is crucial to our emotional regulation). Understanding this is just as important for mothers entering perimenopause or hitting the full menopause, when estrogen levels bounce around erratically before dropping off a cliff. Dealing with sulky teens or young adults who haven't left home while hurtling along on this hormonal rollercoaster can be just as enraging. Same shit, different life stage.

Alongside estrogen, progesterone is another influential hormone in our menstrual cycle and mood. It follows a similar pattern to estrogen throughout the cycle but peaks a bit later, after ovulation. When progesterone breaks down in the body, it produces a by-product called allopregnanolone (let's go with 'allo' for short). So when progesterone is high, in the week or so after ovulation, allo is high. Allo stimulates receptors in the brain for a chemical messenger called GABA. This whole process can have a calming effect, making allo a bit of an 'anti-anxiety hormone', Professor Kulkarni told me. But if conception doesn't happen, then progesterone nosedives. This drop in allo in the week before your period can add agitation and anxiety to the sadness prompted by all the estrogen leaving the building right before the crimson wave hits.

What I didn't know until I was in my 30s was that a not-insignificant number of women experience even more severe symptoms during this time, diagnosed as premenstrual dysphoric disorder (PMDD). Professor Kulkarni said PMDD can affect up to 20 per cent of the menstruating population of reproductive age. Earlier estimates were as low as 2 to 8 per cent but she believes it has been underdiagnosed. As well as standard PMS symptoms like breast tenderness and bloating, PMDD is characterised by severe depression, brain fog, mood swings and rage. And it can come on anywhere in the second half of your cycle, between ovulation and the start of your period. 'Some women describe that for half the cycle, that's half a month, they're dysfunctional, and that's awful because it can go on for decades until she gets to menopause,' Professor Kulkarni told me. 'Some women are living half a life, and it needs to be considered.' PMDD can be something a woman struggles with her whole life, or it can be triggered by a stressor such as the death of a loved one, a divorce or childbirth (and the lack of sleep and hormonal upheaval that follows). However, Professor Kulkarni said, it isn't always immediately apparent and can emerge one or two years postpartum.

To get a diagnosis of PMDD you need to have a marked onset of at least five symptoms over the course of multiple menstrual cycles. These must include at least one core symptom: irritability/anger, tension/anxiety, depressed mood/self-critical thoughts or mood swings, which can include feeling suddenly sad or tearful and increasingly sensitive to rejection. You also need at least one of the following: decreased interest in usual activities, difficulty concentrating, lack of energy, trouble sleeping or sleeping too much, change in appetite, overeating or specific food cravings, a sense of being overwhelmed or out of control, or physical symptoms such as breast tenderness, joint or muscle pain and bloating. There is usually a rapid onset of symptoms in the seven to ten days before bleeding – although this too can vary if the cycle is unpredictable.[4]

At my lowest point I ticked all but one of those symptom boxes, although it took me a long time to put it all together. (Remember, the first step is awareness.) I delayed going back on hormonal contraception for about 18 months after the birth of our second child because I was holding out hope that we might have another. In hindsight I can see that my rage was especially intense at certain points in my cycle.

Hormonal contraception has helped me somewhat, although it's not a magic pill. It can also make things worse, so it's important to ask your doctor about options. One mum I interviewed told me that her first real experience of uncontrollable, inexplicable rage came after starting a progesterone-based pill. 'We had guests over and I was arguing with my partner and I started throwing plates at the kitchen floor. There were children in the house!' she said. Another mum, Louisa, in her late 30s, is unable to take hormonal contraception to manage her PMDD, so awareness is key. 'Now I realise what it is, but at the time I cannot see outside of that,' she told me. 'It's zero patience. Your filter is gone. It's like going from zero to 100 over something as simple as catching your sleeve on the door. I want a divorce every time. And you think, "I didn't feel like this last week."' On reflection, Louisa has a theory that PMDD allows her a window to express exactly what she's feeling: 'I think we have happy hormones the rest of the time. Then all of a sudden I'm not tolerant of the shit … and I go, "This isn't fair." Then a week later I'm back to being a people pleaser.'

Another piece of the hormonal puzzle are these so-called 'happy hormones', like dopamine and serotonin. When these aren't working as well as we need, antidepressants can help. Despite their being a common and successful treatment, I have found myself hesitant to admit here, in black and white, that I have been taking them. I don't want to pathologise all anger in motherhood – we know there are countless social and structural contributors. But anger *can* be a symptom of a number of mental health issues. I was not told this. (Again, awareness …) It wasn't mentioned in the screening questionnaires I took with my GP and obstetrician. The first time I heard another mum draw a link between anger and postpartum depression was in a podcast in 2023, well after I had begun work on this book. Because of that lack of knowledge I didn't think my anger was something I could ask a medical professional about.

In my work as a journalist, I've interviewed women who have suffered severe, life-threatening postnatal depression. They all described a moment when, one day, they could not get out of bed. It wasn't a choice. They just could not make themselves go through the motions anymore. Some were even suicidal. It was such a clear sign that they had reached their breaking point. A sign to themselves, and those around them, that they needed professional, medical help. I often reflected on these interviews and thought, *I'm not like that, so I mustn't be 'bad' enough to need medication.* It wasn't until I reached my own kind of breaking point in 2023 that I realised I wasn't being honest with myself, or anyone else, about how bad I was really feeling. I was getting out of bed, but I was dragging myself out. I dreaded what the day, or the night, would bring. I just wanted to lie there and ignore everything, but I didn't feel I had a choice. So up I rose, on autopilot. And I was angry about it.

The CEO of PANDA (Perinatal Anxiety & Depression Australia), Julie Borninkhof, sees too many parents who wait until things are 'bad enough' to ask for support. 'There's a societal and a cultural normalisation of distress. We're kind of taught to bear it, to suck it up,' Borninkhof, a Melbourne mum of one, told me. 'That construct around "I'm not as bad as the next person" … is a real underminer to us getting what is our right, to be the parents we want to be.' In fact, the earlier people reach out, she said, the easier it usually is to 'help them reframe thinking because it wasn't yet entrenched and they weren't as deep in the negative thoughts'.

It is only now, having asked for help and axed the guilt about needing it, after more than a year on antidepressants and trialling different contraceptives (plus a *whoooooole* lot of work in other areas of my life), that I have the perspective to see how bad it got. I don't think I'll need medication forever, but I wouldn't have got here without it. These days, when I'm woken by a little hand tapping my shoulder or an announcement that someone has wet the bed, I still don't *want* to get out from under the blankets (especially not in winter) but the sense of dread and drudgery is gone. It takes me a moment to come to my senses, but I'm glad to hear a sweet voice at my bedside and pull in a soft little body for a cuddle.

Crying over lost sleep

We might not talk about being angry, but parents talk *a lot* about being tired. There would be almost no one who thinks their night-time routine will not be disrupted by bringing a child into their family. We all know newborns wake a lot. I laughed when my mum told me how she used to sit up in the early hours of the morning to breastfeed me, eating cold upside-down peach cake from the fridge and watching *The Three Stooges* on TV because it was the only thing broadcast at 3 am. (It was the 1980s, remember – no streaming services or smartphones.) We've heard colleagues' tales of sleeping on a sliver of their bed while a toddler lies spread-eagled next to them, or friends army-crawling out of a bedroom once their six-year-old has finally nodded off. Even parents of young adults lose sleep waiting for them to return home from a night out.

I would hate to estimate how many hours of sleep I've lost since I first saw those double lines on a pregnancy test. But someone has done it for me. Dr Oscar Serrallach, who runs a clinic in Byron Bay, New South Wales, and advises the likes of Gwyneth Paltrow on postpartum health, is widely quoted as saying new mums lose an average of 700 hours' sleep in the first year after a baby is born.[1] That works out to just under two hours a night. This may sound like a vast underestimate to some (me included). A large-scale survey of Australian parents in 2024 found 83 per cent of those with kids under five felt sleep deprived at least once a week, and a third were dealing with sleep deprivation every day. The National Parenting Pulse Survey also asked a smaller group of 2000 parents whether being sleep deprived hampered their 'ability to be a calm, loving parent or partner'. (Um, that would be a yes from me.) For two-thirds of those parents it made things 'a little worse', while 16 per cent of mums and dads joined me in the 'a lot worse' camp.[2]

I knew this particular impact of parenting was going to be tough for me. While I could pull all-nighters for work or fun, I've never been good on too little sleep. Pre-kids, if I got less than six solid hours, I would have to eat everything in sight just to stay awake and would want to crash back into bed as soon as I got home that night – where, of course, I would sleep uninterrupted until the alarm went off the next morning. I don't need to set an alarm now. Our children are as regular as clockwork. For most of their early years, they would wake around 5 am. Sometimes 5.15 am or 5.30 am. But if one was still asleep by 6 am, I'd be in a panic that something was wrong. This usually led to me sneaking in to check they were breathing, only to wake them in the process (cue self-directed mum rage). They also aren't the kind of kids who will crawl into bed with us and settle back to sleep for a while. They are the wriggly, chatty type.

I remember the first time our daughter, then a few months old, woke around 2 am and just never went back to sleep. After waving her dad off to work around 6.30 am, I stood in our kitchen thinking, *How am I going to get through the day?* When her brother came along and she was big enough to vacate the cot for him, there was a period where every day started at 2 am. Our big girl was so excited by the novelty of a bed she could simply get out of that if she so much as stirred in the early hours it was game over. Her brother was waking around 2 am for a feed and no sooner would I get him back to sleep than I would hear little feet thudding down the hallway from his sister's room. There was no coaxing her back to sleep, so that was the start of our day. Thankfully, the novelty wore off after a couple of weeks.

There was a particularly brutal period in 2023 when the regular wake-up time inexplicably shifted to 4-something am. I felt like I'd lived an eon by the time I got to the office four hours later. Then, finally, in 2024 there was a drift towards 6 am wake-ups. Again, for no apparent reason. But once or (could I believe it?) *twice* a week I would look at the time on waking to a tap on the arm and realise there was a 6 in front of it!

I have heard there are kids who have to be pried from their beds at 7 am or even 8 am. While I acknowledge this could also trigger some rage if you're running late for school or work, my impulse is to ask these parents where they ordered their model and if they do trade-ins. I have it on good authority that there are also children who don't launch out of bed the second their eyes open, but lie there waiting for their toddler clock to change colour from the blue that signifies night-time to the yellow of the wake-up sun. Our clever daughter understood this concept from the day we bought her such a clock … but took zero notice.

'Darling, is your clock yellow?' I would ask when she appeared in our room, not a hint of daylight peeking through the curtains.

'No,' she would reply simply.

There were attempts to walk her back to her room. Other parents encouraged us to persist: 'It just took a few weeks of being really consistent.' But it took us a couple of years. Until very recently, I still slept with only one earplug in – an attempt to muffle the snoring of my partner next to me while keeping one ear open for a child going bump in the night.

We never enlisted a sleep specialist. Maybe we should have. I know I would have been a less angry mum if I'd been getting more sleep. (While writing this book, if I ever encountered a mum who didn't immediately resonate with the concept of mum rage it was always a woman whose children slept predictably from 7 pm to 7 am.) A part of me kept thinking our kids would 'grow out of it'. Eventually, I came to understand that feeling like I *should* be able to get my kids to sleep better, or for longer, was creating more tension than accepting it just wasn't their thing. (Remember, it's about figuring out what is worth actively resisting and what to let go.) So, if their sleep wasn't going to change, mine had to. (Cue automating my bedtime.) I started getting ready for bed almost straight after the kids. Ideally, I'd be asleep by 8.30 pm. That way, if I was woken at 11 pm or 1 am by a crying toddler or an unsettled preschooler, at least I'd have a few hours under my belt. This routine obviously created a whole lot of other unmet needs – no time for a social life, my partner or working on this book – but the reality was, none of that would have been an option anyway if I wasn't getting enough sleep.

It turns out that keeping a consistent bedtime and wake time is probably one of the most important things you can do for your health. Professor Robert Adams – a respiratory and sleep physician at Flinders Medical Centre and medical director at the Adelaide Institute for Sleep Health at Flinders University – told me that the 'probability that you are asleep at the same time every night' is a stronger predictor of whether you will develop metabolic issues, such as high blood pressure, than how long or how well you sleep for the rest of the night.

As adults we're meant to get between seven and nine hours of sleep, ideally in one uninterrupted block (save for a trip to the toilet, perhaps). During those hours we should be moving through sleep cycles of between 90 and 120 minutes, drifting first into light sleep (stages one and two), then slow-wave or deep sleep, then into the REM (rapid eye movement) stage. 'You get more slow-wave sleep early on [in the night] and more REM sleep later on,' Professor Adams explained. '[This] of course means that disruption at particular times gives you potentially less of one or the other.' Now, why would this be important?

The two latter stages of sleep are where most of the real work happens while we're unconscious. The third stage of a sleep cycle, slow-wave or deep sleep, is when a lot of our cellular repair and regeneration occurs. It is also when the brain clears unnecessary wastes or toxins through the glymphatic system. This, Professor Adams said, is 'a relatively recently recognised function of the brain'. So, let's say you're trying to get eight hours' sleep overnight. Being woken by a hungry baby or an unsettled toddler in the first four hours is more likely to affect these clearing and regenerating processes. This can impact your ability to concentrate and perform complex tasks.

The final stage, REM sleep, is when we dream. Brains scanned during this phase 'look very similar to being awake', Professor Adams said. REM sleep is important for consolidating memories and processing emotions, so we can make a connection between a lack of REM sleep and feeling more irritable or intolerant. Many new mums are rarely getting into this stage. Professor Adams explained, 'If you need a sleep cycle that's 90 or 120 minutes long and you're getting women up sooner than that, it's very hard to get the full cycle, so you're probably not getting out of stage two sleep very much. If you think of that mother who is always being woken up like that and never getting to the end of the cycle ... they are deprived of a lot of REM sleep. That mechanism around emotional regulation and emotional memory, working out what we thought of the day before ... just doesn't ever happen.'

At this point in our conversation I asked, jokingly, just how serious these missing hours are. Like, is the terrible sleep I've had since becoming a mum shortening my life? Professor Adams, who has three grown-up children, gave me a sheepish shrug as if to say, 'Well, yeah, kind of.' (Months later, I come across an alarming American study showing that consistently getting less than seven hours of sleep a night in the six months after a baby is born did in fact take years off a group of 33 mothers' lives.[3] Well, it accelerated their biological age, anyway.) I might feel like death after a rough night with the kids, but Professor Adams reassured me that the more realistic short-term implications are brain fog, irritability and food cravings. 'Your brain doesn't work as well ... and everything literally just slows down.'

We already know that lack of sleep was overwhelmingly identified in the Angry Mums Club as the top factor contributing to their anger. A series of studies by Canadian researchers has unearthed links between poor sleep and postpartum anger. In 2022, the results of a survey of 278 Canadian mothers of babies aged six to 12 months showed that half of the mothers rated their sleep as poor, almost a third reported feelings of intense anger and a quarter exhibited symptoms of probable depression. (Among the angry mums the rate of probable depression was almost half.) The authors found that women who perceived their sleep as fairly bad or very bad were almost three times more likely to feel anger than those who felt their sleep was fairly good or very good. Having multiple children (and so more chance of being woken) also increased the likelihood of feeling angry.[4]

In another paper, 'Seeing red', about the women we heard of earlier who scored highly on short-term anger, the same researchers found the need for adequate sleep was the 'most consistently compromised physical need [among mothers] that increased feelings of being on edge and intense anger'.[5] In an extremely validating sentence for those of us in the Angry Mums Club, the authors described intense anger as 'a relevant mood disturbance in the postpartum period' and noted sleep difficulties 'significantly contribute to women's anger after childbirth'.[6]

An American study of 142 adults (not necessarily parents) looked at the effect of accruing a sleep debt over just two days and found it 'universally intensified anger'. Participants were either allowed to sleep as normal or restricted to five or six hours a night. Their anger was tested by exposing them to two types of noise: one that sounded like spraying water and a louder static signal that proved to be more provoking. (There is an irony here that white noise was used to intentionally irritate sleep-deprived adults, and yet it is the same kind of noise that millions of parents rely on to lull their babies to sleep.) In short, this 2019 study showed that losing sleep is likely to 'make a person angrier under irritating conditions'.[7] Um ... yep.

I know there are mums out there who rise from their warm bed in the middle of the night to tend to crying, thirsty, hungry, bed-wetting children calmly and repeatedly. I'm calm the first time. And the second. But repeated wake-ups when it's pitch dark outside, night after night, are a sure-fire trigger for my mum rage. I wanted to know why it feels so much harder to control when the lights are out, so I approached clinical psychologist and sleep expert Professor Sarah Blunden, who has worked with hundreds of families through her Paediatric Sleep Clinic. She is also the head of paediatric sleep research at Central Queensland University, founder of the Australian Centre for Education in Sleep, and co-author of *The Sensible Sleep Solution*. During a phone interview on a day of back-to-back meetings, Professor Blunden told me that while very few mothers would ever admit that they're angry because their child doesn't sleep, the proportion of those she has worked with who are 'frustrated' by their situation would be at least 90 per cent. 'That frustration can lead to anger,' she told me, 'and it's very, very common.'

We learned earlier about the brain circuitry of anger. Our amygdalae, which are part of the limbic system, set off our threat warning system and often act before our prefrontal cortex has a chance to intervene with some common sense. Professor Blunden told me that the prefrontal cortex is the part of the brain that actually needs the most sleep to function properly. It needs a 'hibernation of sorts' overnight. 'If you don't get the sleep that you need, your prefrontal cortex won't react the way that it should,' she said. 'If you perceive danger or threat or stress, your amygdalae will respond. It will take over the focus and you won't be able to think straight. You start thinking, "My baby's woken up, here I am again, this has happened ten times a night." You haven't got the thinking capacity to say, "Now stop, it's okay."'

And it is worse when we're woken out of a period of deep sleep. We get more of this type of sleep in the first half of the night when, as Professor Blunden pointed out, 'melatonin, our sleep hormone, is the highest, so you will be groggier. It's very, very, very difficult for us to wake up because our body is in the deepest sleep.' Conversely, if we're in the light stage of sleep, we're likely to wake very quickly or think we haven't been asleep at all.

There is another reason why it can all feel so much harder at night. If you've raised little kids, you're surely familiar with the feeling that settles over a household when it's dark and muted outside. I have beautiful memories of breastfeeding my babies, nestled in a rocking chair, the room dimly lit by a lamp. I can picture their rosebud lips and flushed cheeks as they fell into the serene sleep that came with a full belly. But it could also be lonely. I often used to look out the window, as if the streetlights could keep me company, wondering how long the night would last. It turns out there's a biological reason why it feels darkest before the dawn and it has to do with our circadian rhythm. This is our internal clock, which, when it's working well, ensures our body regulates hormones like melatonin to rise in the evening so we feel sleepy, and cortisol to rise in the morning so we wake. But Professor Blunden told me something that kind of blew my mind. Every cell in our body has its own circadian rhythm and this doesn't just affect when we sleep, but how we feel at different times of the day. 'Melatonin, which kicks in at night-time and makes us sleep, has a chemical pathway that interacts with dopamine and serotonin, which are our happy hormones,' she said. 'So if melatonin is disrupted, the happy hormones are disrupted too and our mood is worse.' (It's not just in my head then ...)

I also talked to Professor Jayashri Kulkarni, the psychiatrist we heard from in the previous chapter, about the impact hormones have on our sleep and mood. 'Sleep deprivation is a very underrated stressor because all the hormones that should be nicely settling with a good seven hours' sleep are not,' she said. One of the key hormones that needs a good rest to reset is cortisol. Professor Kulkarni explained that the broken sleep often experienced by mothers means we don't get a daily rhythm of 'morning, afternoon, evening, but it's all one blurry mess'. This wreaks havoc on cortisol production, which has wide-ranging effects on other processes in the body, including our stress response and metabolism. Estrogen, central to our menstrual cycle, is also important in regulating sleep. 'When there are wild fluctuations in estrogen, that's when sleep goes off,' she said. 'You see this in the first trimester of pregnancy, a very common time for sleep just to disappear because there's suddenly a big rise in estrogen. And you see it in menopause as well' – a time when estrogen drops.

All of these variables can contribute to a feeling of dread as each night approaches. *Will my kid sleep? Will I sleep?* Professor Blunden sees many mothers who develop a fear of not being able to nod off. 'You actually can't relax,' she said. 'You think, "What's going to happen tonight?"' Over time this can become an automatic reaction and mums develop 'almost a trauma response' to the slightest indication that it is going to be a rough night. 'You might hear a murmur from the baby and you go, "See, it's gonna happen again",' Professor Blunden said, as if reading a printout of my inner monologue most evenings in the early 2020s. For this reason, there are significant benefits in treating mothers for insomnia 'over and above their child's sleep problems', she said. 'To get mum good sleep will be a contributor to everything. The prefrontal cortex can problem-solve better … the amygdala is not so sensitive, so you can be less irritable.' Getting good sleep in your household might require asking for help from an expert or a babysitter, actively resisting the calls from a child's bedroom or axing the guilt about waiting to see if they nod off on their own.

The reality in our household is that I do 90 per cent of the night-time duty. I used to fume at my partner's ability to sleep through a child calling out. Because it was me rising repeatedly to feed them when they were babies, an expectation was set that it would be me they saw when they woke. Now, if my partner does wake up, his attempts to take a child calling out for me back to bed usually just inflame the situation. (We'll talk more about what contributes to this infuriating 'default parent' situation in a later chapter.) Again, other parents have urged us to persist, telling us we could break the habit. But to be honest, I'm too tired and cranky to break habits at 2 am. I just want the fastest route back to the land of Nod. So some nights I deliver a not-so-gentle 'back to bed' at increasing volumes. And on others I take a world tour of our home, sleeping at some point in every bed in the house.

While I wish it was different, it's not uncommon. Analysis of Australian parents' sleep patterns in 2021 found while mums got a little less sleep than childless women, for dads there was 'no evidence that having children of any age' meant they lost sleep.[8] A 2016 paper by researchers at the University of Queensland, titled 'Doing gender overnight', also examined how differently Australian mums and dads fare in the sleep stakes. Becoming a parent costs a person almost 1.5 hours of sleep a week, compared to non-parents, they found. That increases to almost four hours by the third child. The news is worst for mums, who experience 'significantly lower sleep quality' than dads until their youngest child turns four, 'when they finally catch up'. During the child's first year, dads sleep an average of almost three hours more than mums each week. If you're a single mum you're really losing out, sleeping an average four hours less than your partnered peers. The sleep loss is, of course, from waking to tend to children's needs, but the researchers also found that parents' sleep time was further eroded by having to do paid work or household tasks, or taking time for 'leisure activities', after children went to bed.[9]

Clinical psychologist Dr Nicole Williams works with a lot of mums struggling with a lack of sleep. And she knows how hard it is – her first baby 'woke up screaming ten-plus times a night for a year and a half'. However, I got a bit of a reality check when I interviewed her at her Adelaide office. As I listened back to the recording of our conversation, I could still hear the bewilderment in my voice as Dr Williams told me I had a *choice*. 'If it's one o'clock in the morning, the baby's woken for the fourth time and I'm the one who's responding, there can very easily be a lot of anger towards a partner who's still asleep, towards the baby for being awake,' she said, as I nodded in furious agreement. But she asked me to consider how I could 'change the way I relate to those experiences'. I could choose not to get up. I could choose to put ear plugs in. I could choose to go and sleep in a different place, she offered. I remember looking at her, my mouth agape, wanting to say, '*What* choice?!' Is my choice to lie there and listen to my kid howl? Is my choice to elbow my partner in the ribs and then still have to listen to the kid howl while he takes a while to wake up and a while longer to settle them? Apparently, yes. 'So much of that is values driven,' Dr Williams said. 'We're making a decision that that's the sort of parent that we want to be. It is not my preference to be awake, but it is my preference to respond.'

There is a moment of silence on the recording after Dr Williams dropped the choice bomb on me. She's right, of course. The kind of parent I want to be is one who meets my child's needs. But often it doesn't *feel* like a choice. And that's the problem. 'If you feel like you don't have a choice then you feel angry,' she acknowledged. 'Or helpless, which makes us feel angry. Or anxious ... or that there's injustice, which also makes me feel angry. If we get caught up in those ways of thinking, even unconsciously, we're in a very different headspace and we can get very frustrated.' Instead, Dr Williams encourages us to adopt a 'beginner's mind' and consider each challenge as if it is the first time we've experienced it. 'Objectively, there's not a huge amount different at the fifth wake-up a night as the first wake-up, but it feels different,' she said. 'The frustration is mainly that I shouldn't be awake, and that's perceived as a threat, which then goes to anger.' If, instead, we can treat every sleep interruption like it's the first interruption of the night – or for that matter, every time a child doesn't listen, has a tantrum or talks back – then it can prolong our patience. 'I talk to women about having a volcano of "stuff" [inside them] and anger is really the point that the volcano is exploding,' Dr Williams told me. Adopting a beginner's mindset helps to 'bring that lava back down so we can tolerate more before we're at that point'.

What we're really talking about here is mindfulness. But, honestly, every time I hear that word I have to stifle an involuntary eye roll. It appears to be the answer to almost everything but also feels so vague. It can be anything from pausing to 'ground yourself' while your teenager is ranting that you're ruining their life, to dropping into a lotus pose for 20 minutes every night before bed (after writing in your gratitude journal, of course). Yet when I stop to think about Dr Williams' example, it is actually more tangible and specific than many others I've heard. I'm not sure I could go so far as to convince myself that every time the toddler cries for mummy or the preschooler wants *another* snack before bed it actually *is* the first time. But telling myself 'I handled it the first time, I can handle it again because I want to be there for my child' might help more than telling myself to take a bloody deep breath.

Hangry mum

It was 1.37 am and I was standing next to the microwave, baby cradled in one arm, muffin clutched in my other hand. I can still remember the taste of that muffin, made for me by my cousin who has three children about a decade older than mine. It had dark chocolate chips, coconut, raspberries and a hint of lemon. It was warm from being defrosted in the microwave and just the right combination of carbs, fat and sugar. As I inhaled that perfect one-handed snack in our darkened kitchen, bathed in the glow of the microwave's internal light, I could feel my tension receding.

Minutes earlier, I had been upstairs trying to rock our firstborn back to sleep after a night-time feed. With every push on the rocking chair, I had been growing more impatient ... and hangry. Eventually, I couldn't hold off any longer. I'd launched myself out of the chair, baby still wide awake in the crook of my arm, and scurried downstairs to retrieve the muffin from the freezer. It was all I had been able to think about for the past 15 minutes. Waiting for the seconds to count down on the microwave timer had been agony. Finally, it beeped, signalling my treat was ready for consumption. In less than 30 seconds it was chewed and swallowed, and by the time it hit my stomach the world began to seem manageable again. I glugged some water and headed back upstairs. I can't say how long it took to get my daughter back to sleep after that, but the fact is it wouldn't have mattered anywhere near as much by then. With a full stomach I could withstand the tedium once more.

Why does being hungry make us irritable? Why does it feel at times like we can do nothing else, think about nothing else, until we eat? For me, hunger is right up there with lack of sleep when it comes to mum rage triggers. Motherhood, especially in the early stages, creates a perfect storm in which we have less time to eat, cook or organise nutritious or satisfying meals. We're eating at odd hours, too busy to eat or bingeing at the end of the day once we finally have a moment to ourselves. Almost one in five Angry Mums Club members said their anger was triggered by hunger, and two in five felt poor nutrition contributed to their irritable mood.

The feeling of being hangry – a portmanteau of hungry and angry – has been validated in research, including the findings of a study of 64 Europeans who tracked their hunger and emotions five times a day for three weeks. The authors of the 'Hangry in the field' paper concluded that 'the experience of being hangry is real'. The feeling of hunger was associated among the participants with increased anger and irritability, and reduced pleasure. These findings remained stable even when age, sex, body mass index, eating behaviours and the participants' usual tendencies towards anger were taken into account. The authors also noted other studies that have shown that low blood sugar levels, which happen when we don't eat for a while, can lead to greater impulsivity, anger and aggression.[1]

As Dr Mansi Dass Singh, a registered nutritionist and biomedical science lecturer, explained to me, sugar (or glucose) levels in the blood are monitored in the brain by the hypothalamus, as well as other glands around the body that make up our endocrine system. Remember the hypothalamus? The tiny gland in our brain that monitors basic functions like our heart rate, breathing and digestion. When it senses our blood sugar levels are low, alarm bells start ringing. It's an evolutionary signal that our brain perceives as a threat. *We won't last too long without food; better do something about that quick smart.* To spur us into action, the body produces the stress hormone cortisol, and another hormone called glucagon, which does the groundwork of retrieving glucose stores in the body. 'The way cortisol talks to the brain is it aggravates our sympathetic nervous system to fight, and that can lead to irritation,' Dr Dass Singh told me over the phone. 'The way we have evolved, we have this conditioning that whenever we are low [in blood sugar] we go into a fight or flight mode. *Something is not right. I don't have food. I'm under threat.*' Rationally, we know there is a fridge full of food downstairs and we can go and eat whatever we want after the baby finally falls asleep, but our brain is jumping ahead. *What if it takes too long? What if we die of starvation in the meantime? That won't do. Better give this mum a prod to get her moving towards that fridge.*

This drive often seems impossible for me to ignore. My early solution was to stash muesli bars in every room of our house so if I was nap-trapped under a baby, or one of the kids took longer to settle than anticipated, I was never far from instant sustenance. (I now give every new mum non-perishable snacks in a survival pack at my first visit after their baby is born.) The dinner/bedtime juggle was harder to negotiate. In an ideal world I would have liked to have, say, seven minutes of peace and quiet to eat my dinner uninterrupted at the end of the day. This meant for a long time I would wait until my partner and I had fed and settled the kids to sleep, because if they are conscious and I am visible it is pretty difficult to achieve peace or quiet. 'What's that, Mum? Is that chicken? Is that your chicken? Is that your yummy chicken on your plate, Mummy? Can I try some?'

Some nights, bedtime would go smoothly and I'd be sitting at our dining table eating a hot meal by 7.30 pm. Other nights it would drag out until 8 pm or 8.30 pm and all I would be thinking about was my bowl of pasta congealing on the kitchen bench. Or worse, what I was going to cook for dinner when I finally got back downstairs. I would get so impatient, so hangry, and the mum rage would boil over in rushing and snapping. So now I eat earlier with the kids, amid the chaos, or have a late afternoon snack to get me through. Less peace and quiet while I'm eating, but usually a more peaceful bedtime.

Unfortunately, scarfing down food in whatever fashion we can has become a hallmark of mothering. American mum of four and Postpartum University founder Maranda Bower knows this well. 'I think the hangry feeling is something that so many of us can relate to,' she told me over a video call from her home in Alaska. 'We feel it often in motherhood because we forget ourselves. We're so busy. When we do find ourselves eating something, it's got to be fast. It's that couple of potato chips or the leftover chicken nuggets from our toddler. We're able to put [our hunger] on the backburner and not even notice it. And then it overflows ... you explode, the anger, the rage really comes out.'

It was her experience of mum rage, as well as postpartum depression, anxiety and panic attacks, that prompted Bower to delve into the importance of nutrition for mothers, especially in the months after birth. What she learned drove her to establish Postpartum University, which educates professionals who work with people giving birth to understand what their body needs and the best way to get it. 'Our bodies feel really different during this time, but nobody is teaching us ... what's going on,' she told me.

I took the video call with Bower in our laundry, of all places, because it was the only room in our open-plan home where I could conduct an interview at 4.30 am (due to the time difference) and not wake our children. I heard the first little footsteps running down the hall about four minutes after we hung up at 5.15 am. When I asked Bower to describe her experience of mum rage to me, she said it felt 'uncontrollable ... I didn't feel at the time that there was any sort of rhyme or reason to it. I felt like I was out of my body, that it wasn't really me, and I would go into a rage on my family. I would be fine, cooking in the kitchen ... then somebody spills a cup of water all over the floor and all of a sudden there was this anger. I would tell myself, "What are you doing? This is not okay, stop yelling at your kids." But I couldn't stop.' She described a 'rollercoaster of emotions' that would follow. 'We focus on the rage, but we forget all of the other emotions that come with it as well, that are just as damaging. You've got the guilt, you've got the shame, you've got the fear, like if this is possible within me, what else is possible? Am I going to scar my children for life? I definitely thought that I was very, very alone in everything that I was experiencing.'

It is remarkable how much of an impact what we eat has on what we think. Science has now shown that what ends up in our gut plays a role in determining how well we are able to produce hormones like serotonin and dopamine, which directly affect our brain and emotional state. As nutritionist Dr Dass Singh explained, certain gut bacteria are key. She gave the example of fibre. Usually, when we eat a vegetable like broccoli or cauliflower, we eat the florets but maybe not the stem. But it is the stem that has the fibre our good gut bacteria need. 'Good bacteria are able to digest and ferment that fibre and convert it to some short-chain fatty acids,' she told me. The main one, butyrate, 'keeps our gut healthy' because it acts as fuel for the cells in our colon. Some species of good gut bacteria also produce serotonin, one of those 'happy hormones'. 'If the gut is happy then it is able to communicate to the brain that I am happy and make possible the release of happy mood neurotransmitters, like serotonin,' Dr Dass Singh said.

Now, I know, it's hard enough to maintain a balanced diet when you're child-free with disposable income and time to yourself, let alone with a child hanging off each leg the minute you get home from work and search the freezer for something to reheat. To be clear, I am *not* about to give any kind of diet advice. I'm also not here to give medical advice, but I wanted to better understand how some key nutrients (or lack of them) could be messing with my mood.

In *The Postnatal Depletion Cure*, Dr Oscar Serrallach describes what he terms 'postnatal depletion syndrome': a collection of symptoms many mothers experience in the years after giving birth. He argues that key nutrients are depleted during pregnancy, postpartum and breastfeeding, and not replaced to high enough levels, which can affect our energy and mood.[2]

Iron is at the top of this list, particularly because it carries oxygen around the body and is crucial in the process of turning macronutrients in food into fuel for energy. Irritability and trouble concentrating are often listed as symptoms of anaemia, or iron deficiency.[3] Many women need iron supplementation during pregnancy due to making all that extra blood for the baby. Iron is also passed on to babies during breastfeeding, and it is depleted again when, or if, our period returns. It is found in highest concentrations in organ meat and red meat, as well as dark leafy green vegetables. Dr Dass Singh warns there are a few traps we can fall into that mean we might be getting less iron than we think. For iron to do its work properly, it needs to be consumed with vitamin C, so make sure you've got some tomato or capsicum on your beef burger. But try to steer clear of drinking coffee, tea or (sigh) a glass of wine with your steak or meatloaf. These beverages contain caffeine, tannins, phenols or phytates, which bind to iron and stop it being properly absorbed. Same goes for a café latte or big bowl of cereal and milk with your iron supplement in the morning: calcium binds with iron to make an insoluble compound that your body simply sends through your gut and out the other end.

Next up, *magnesium*, which Dr Dass Singh told me is necessary for about 300 enzymes in your body to work properly. It is most commonly used in making proteins, like skin or hair (for yourself or a foetus), working muscles and turning fuel into energy. All this means it can be easily depleted. Dr Serrallach, meanwhile, noted that stress causes us to lose more magnesium through our urine. He added that magnesium is important in producing melatonin (to help us sleep) and releasing happy hormone neurotransmitters.[4] It is found in higher concentrations in dark green leafy vegetables, legumes, nuts, seeds and whole grains but is also easy and relatively cheap to supplement with tablets.

To round out this short list, *omega-3 fatty acids* and *vitamin D* both play a role in helping to manage inflammation in the body. A little bit of inflammation is necessary, Dr Dass Singh says, to send a message when we are hurt, but too much can cause problems. The evidence is mixed but there is a growing body of research that suggests chronic inflammation can be associated with mental states like depression. Levels of omega-3 fatty acids (like those in oily fish) have been found to be low in depressed patients.[5] Dr Dass Singh says vitamin D also supports our immune cells 'to transform into the shining knights' that bolster our immune system and curb inflammation. Sunlight is a good source of vitamin D, as are fatty fish, eggs, activated mushrooms and beef liver.

And although it's not a nutrient, we should also mention sleep again here. As well as affecting our ability to concentrate and regulate our emotions, sleep deprivation affects our appetite and food cravings. Proper sleep helps our body regulate hormones, including ghrelin (which signals hunger) and leptin (which tells us we're full). Sleep expert Professor Robert Adams broke it down really simply for me: 'When people have relatively less sleep, they tend to make poor food choices.' At that point in our conversation, I felt like he must have been standing in my kitchen in my early days of parenting. However, he followed up with a sentence that made me feel better: 'It's a real thing and overcoming that requires a substantial amount of effort.' Automating can be very helpful here. Online grocery ordering systems enable you to select the same set of items you bought the week before. So stack that list with helpful, tasty options then rinse and repeat. Or maybe a meal delivery service would take the pressure off for a bit (a great group present idea for a baby shower). And don't forget to ask for help: if people are coming to visit you and your new baby, ask them to bring lunch, or something to pop in the freezer, instead of flowers.

You might want to ask your GP a few questions about all this. Just because you're feeling irritable or angry doesn't mean you're necessarily deficient in any particular nutrient, but if you think it's contributing to your mum rage it can't hurt to find out. Australia's healthcare system enables GPs to order basic blood tests with no out-of-pocket cost to the patient. Dr Dass Singh said routine checks can measure levels of iron, folate, vitamin D and vitamin B12. And if you want to investigate further, a clinical nutritionist or dietician can look at the 'bigger picture'.

Western culture is still, in many ways, playing catch-up to Eastern philosophies when it comes to the importance of food to our health, both physical and mental. The time just after birth has long been recognised in countries like China and India as crucial for eating well and resting. Dr Dass Singh was living in Delhi, India, when she had her son, now in his mid-20s, and for the first week after the birth her female relatives restricted her to a diet of milk, nuts, ghee, turmeric and caraway seeds – to provide fats, fight inflammation and encourage breastmilk production. She would like to see more exploration of the science behind these cultural practices.

The thing I craved most after my daughter was born was a fresh ham sandwich. After the birth of our son, my partner brought a platter of soft cheeses and cured meats to the hospital. When we returned home, both times, my cousin brought around a batch of *those* muffins. There were also chicken and vegetable patties delivered by an aunty, which provided a balanced meal for everyone including our toddler. And after we all got Covid for the first time, my best friend's mum dropped some soup at our door. My mother-in-law always goes to the effort of making something gluten-free that I can eat at celebration meals. And my mum sends us home from Sunday night dinner at their place with a fridge full of leftovers. There are so many women who have shared food with me in this way since I became a mum. And if that isn't a real-life example of the adage 'food is love', I don't know what is.

Pain in the ... everything

Parenting is a pain. The pain started in my hips and groin around 14 weeks into my first pregnancy and hasn't really let up. Back aches, stretching skin ... then the prick of a needle to induce labour and it really kicked up a gear. We've all watched that movie scene where the mother in labour screams at her partner or her doctor. Instinctively, we know there must be a link between pain and anger because we feel it. We stub our toe, we let out an expletive. A headache makes us irritable. Our pain pathways are a complicated area of science, and everyone reacts differently, but there is enough understanding in the field now to reassure us that the impact of pain on our mood is real.

I will never forget the unique intensity of those first labour cramps. Or the moment, just before both my children were born, when I regretted not asking for the epidural. I didn't have to contend with recovery from a C-section, episiotomy or serious tears, but after the happy hormones began to wear off everything ached. My chest went rock hard and then we struggled to figure out breastfeeding. I can still remember clenching in anticipation each time I guided a hungry little mouth to latch, knowing it would hurt like hell.

Parenting is manual labour. All that bending to get a baby in and out of their cot. Strapping them to your body like you're training for some ultra-endurance event with a weighted vest. The side-to-side rock that ruined my knees, already pushed to their limit by the weight of carrying a human in my guts for nine months. The swing to shush them to sleep that leaves your arms quivering like jelly. Then there's the specific muscles recruited to change a nappy when they're in that rolling-like-a-crocodile stage. Or lugging your toddler through the car park because otherwise they will stand there and cry at oncoming traffic.

Eventually, parenting becomes less physical. Kids can walk and wipe their own bums and climb into their own beds. But there are plenty of reasons mums continue to carry pain. The effects of birth trauma or a decimated pelvic floor can be long-lasting. Each month we may have to reach for the painkillers when (or if) our period returns. Children are germ factories, and gastro and the flu hurt too. As does copping an elbow to the face or having your hair pulled by a dysregulated kid (as more than one Angry Mums Club member reported). Stress (and yelling) creates tension and headaches. And many women are living with chronic illness or conditions that make everyday life painful. For example, the 2025 Jean Hailes National Women's Health Survey found one in three Australian women suffer from migraines. Among them, half experienced more than one a week and almost two-thirds said they were severe or very severe.[1]

For me, it's endometriosis, a condition that affects one in seven women.[2] Endo, as it's known by those who have it, causes tissue similar to the lining of the uterus to grow elsewhere in the body and can induce a wide range of symptoms including cramps, bloating and abdominal pain, nausea, fatigue, nerve pain, inflammation, bladder irritation, body aches and discomfort during sex or while going to the toilet. It can also lead to organ damage or fertility difficulties. Many sufferers are told, pre-diagnosis, that it is irritable bowel syndrome, a food intolerance, stress ... or that being uncomfortable is just part of being a woman. On most days endo causes me some level of discomfort, pain or stiffness. My wick is shorter, my threshold is lower. It can usually be managed by taking ibuprofen and swapping my skinny jeans for track pants, but on the bad days it can hurt to sit down, even slowly, because connecting with the seat sends a vibration up through my ovaries. An unexpected sneeze can be disastrous. Sometimes there are stabbing pains or muscle spasms. Often the most debilitating symptoms are the fatigue and nausea. I feel like I want to throw up and fall into bed, but that's not always an option when you're responsible for kids. My worst endo day since becoming a mum happened when I was home alone with a toddler and a baby. It took everything I had (including the strong pain meds) to get us all in the car and head to the refuge of my parents' house. They distracted the kids, and I got up to go to the loo but promptly dropped to the kitchen floor with a stab of pain up the right side of my back. I don't know what I would have done if I didn't have a safe place to go for help. (More on the importance of the village later.)

While writing this chapter, I opened an internet search engine and typed in 'why does physical pain ...' Before I could finish typing my sentence, the algorithm suggested '... make me angry' among the most commonly searched phrases. It's a complicated question, scientists don't have all the answers and everyone has a unique sensitivity, but there is research that links the experience of pain with increased aggression and poor mood.

Work by UNSW Sydney and NeuRA scientists has found people with chronic pain have an imbalance of neurotransmitters, which can affect the way the brain regulates emotions. A 2019 study reported people with persistent pain had low levels of the neurotransmitter glutamate, which impaired their ability to manage feelings of fear, worry and negative thinking.[3] In a 2021 study, researchers found persistent pain was also associated with a drop in the neurotransmitter GABA, which we learned earlier can have a calming effect. The team scanned the brains of 24 people with chronic pain and 24 without, and found that the participants in pain also had lower levels of GABA.[4] In a media release about those findings, senior author, neuroscientist and psychologist Professor Sylvia Gustin said the studies showed chronic pain has a real effect on our brains and our ability to regulate our emotions.[5]

Short, sharp pain can also make us more hostile. Chinese researchers in 2023 found that inducing acute pain in study participants made them more aggressive when given the chance to retaliate against people who judged them – regardless of whether the feedback was positive or negative. The authors posited this could have been because the experience of pain drew 'cognitive resources' to parts of the brain registering pain and away from areas that assess and react to other information in the environment, such as social cues.[6]

There is a key part of the brain involved here, called the salience network.[7] As the name suggests, it's involved in directing attention to what is important and filtering distractions. It prioritises things that are emotionally charged, new or key to our survival. Given that pain can have serious consequences, it is perceived as very important by the salience network and will usually be prioritised (diverting cognitive resources, as it were). But the salience network *can* manage scenarios where there are competing demands, such as enabling us to continue to run away from a sabre-toothed tiger after we have sprained our ankle.

There is also overlap in the parts of the brain activated by physical pain and emotional pain or social rejection.[8] This doesn't mean our brain can't tell them apart, and some scientists contest how strong the overlap is, but a number of studies have shown that we process both types of pain in the same regions of the brain. And there is some evidence of the reverse, that social or emotional pain can influence our perception of physical pain. For example, one study found people reported more pain when exposed to heat if they also felt more socially excluded.[9]

It's not a stretch to conclude that mums who feel unsupported by their partners, family or social networks may feel their bodily pain is worse, and in turn their mood can sour. Indeed the former head of Pain Australia Giulia Jones told me pain is influenced by how comfortable, connected and supported you feel. 'So let's say you're going down the pain spectrum and … you have no support, you'll report a higher number on your pain score than if you have social support, which makes you feel like you're going to be okay,' Jones, a mum of six, explained from her office in Canberra. We've all been there, right? Those days when we're in the trenches alone with the kids – maybe it was a Covid lockdown, or the weather was too bad to get out and see anyone, or the whole family caught gastro. That feeling of isolation, or frustration, can seep into your bones. Or show up as a headache or a stomach ache.

Laura, an Adelaide mum of three, also has endo, as well as fibromyalgia and osteoarthritis. 'The pain feels worse when I look around and no one else is doing anything,' she told me. 'I think, "You're not in pain, why aren't you helping?" I've been in pain so long now that I kind of take it in my stride, but some days that is harder. I'm more tired, my temper is shorter and I'm angry at myself that I can't handle it. Then there's the guilt, feeling so terrible that I've just snapped at everyone and then around we go again in the cycle.' Laura, who is in her 40s, gave me an example of a common evening in her household. The teenagers are sitting on the couch while Laura is nearby in the kitchen. 'They can hear me grunting in pain as I move and they might look up from their phones and think, *Oh yeah, there she goes*. Meanwhile, I'm making dinner for them, I'm setting the table and no one else in this house is doing anything. But they're all very hungry.' Other times, Laura said, it is watching kids make a mess and realising 'I will have to clean that up'. Just thinking about all the bending that will be involved is painful.

I felt the same way when my three-year-old gave me 'that look' just before he would take off, running away from me in a shopping centre. I knew I was going to have to chase him down and pick him up. He's a strong little fella and can wriggle for Australia, so I knew it was going to hurt. Before anything had even happened, I was agitated. Same with trying to get kids into car seats. There is a moment, after they're all buckled in, when I lean against the closed door and sigh as the impact of all that twisting and pulling starts to bubble up in my lower back and abdomen. That moment before I have to open the driver's door, let out the crying or squealing that I had momentarily silenced inside, and get on with the day. Getting kids in the car should be added as the next Olympic sport.

There are about 1.7 million Australian women living with persistent pain.[10] Like Laura and me, Giulia Jones is among them. In early secondary school she injured her coccyx when another student pulled a chair out from underneath her. She has since carried six children to term, and birthed them by Caesarean section. While the recovery from surgery was painful, it was the sitting for hours on end nursing that really aggravated her existing injury. 'If I had a more comfortable pillow under my butt when I was breastfeeding, I might have actually been a less distressed mother. By the time I had my fifth baby, I made my husband go and buy a really comfortable breastfeeding chair,' she told me with a laugh.

Jones, a former Liberal MP in the Australian Capital Territory Parliament, now has a custom pillow she takes with her in the car and to work. She also reminds mums they don't need to soldier on if taking some paracetamol might make the day infinitely easier to manage. But she acknowledges it took her a long time to 'come to terms with the underlying pain I was living with most days of my life. I was getting distressed because I hadn't quite registered – not only was the baby crying distressing me, but my chronic pain was distressing me,' she explained. 'It's a bit like if you had a fringe that was too long and you can't see, right? You might be used to it but it's affecting everything you do. A lot of new mums are living right on the edge of that limit anyway when you've got a baby that needs you 24 hours a day, seven days a week ... because the body has been stretched and used and exhausted. And then if you're not acknowledging and not understanding that you have a pain condition, that is enough to tip anybody over the edge.'

Grief and loss

Anger is recognised as one of the five major stages of the grieving process, and so many women are grappling with grief while mothering. It could be the death of a parent, partner, sibling or friend. They may have experienced abortion, pregnancy loss, stillbirth, medical termination or the death of a child through accident or illness. Among the random 200 mums I surveyed for this book alone, there were at least nine grieving a loss. One said the death of her baby had made her 'wild with grief'. Some mums who have lost a child have told me it completely doused their fury, as they were simply grateful to have surviving or later children to tend to, no matter how demanding or difficult their behaviour might be. But many are furious with the unfairness of their loss, and rightly so. Yet they are shamed and judged for feeling, and expressing, this rage.

Meira's daughter Neave only lived for eight days after her birth. She was delivered by emergency Caesarean section after her heart stopped beating just as her mother began to push. It took 11 terrifying minutes for doctors to pull Neave from Meira's womb, and another nine excruciating minutes to resuscitate her. While doctors were working on Neave, Meira began to haemorrhage and had to be put under a general anaesthetic. She didn't see her daughter for two days. 'It took me a while to really understand what had happened,' she told me, years later. We met at a suburban library on a cool afternoon towards the end of winter. Clutching decaffeinated coffees, we were the only ones in the quiet room and our voices echoed off the floorboards. Meira, her husband Andrew and their firstborn Ari were in Australia visiting family – a long plane ride from where they live overseas. She had agreed to spend part of her precious time here with me because hers is a story that cannot be grasped over email or video call.

'On TV, with an emergency C-section, you think it's two minutes later and the baby is born, but it's not,' Meira told me. For Neave, 'it was eleven minutes. And it was just too long. The regions of her brain that had lesions on them were in her brain stem, which is all your base functions, breathing, reflexes and swallowing.' Doctors put Neave into a hypothermic coma to reduce her core body temperature, which has been shown to save brain function. 'But it wasn't enough,' Meira said, tears spilling down her cheeks.

Neave was born on a Tuesday. By Wednesday evening Meira was stable enough to be transferred to the hospital where her daughter was being treated. On the Saturday doctors told Meira and Andrew that Neave's 'condition was incompatible with life'. They began to scale back her care, especially anything that might be causing pain, like the blood pressure cuff regularly squeezing her tiny arm. Meira's mum had booked the first flight over from Australia but was still days away.

Eventually, the time came. 'We'd spent four days with the really clear knowledge that she was going to die,'

Meira explained shakily. 'That last day she had started to deteriorate. I got to hold her and they took out the tube.' Her voice caught as more tears spilled. 'It took a really long time [for her] to die. We stayed with her for a while after because we never really got to see her face because she was covered in tubes. You don't want to leave.'

In the months afterwards Meira struggled to get out of bed. When her mum managed to coax her out for a walk she would find herself saying 'mean things' to her. She also directed her grief at Ari, who was about two and a half at the time. 'I had so little to give that if he didn't follow instructions immediately I would snap at him. I had no fuse,' Meira said, adding she felt awful about this in hindsight. 'None of this was his fault. It's this shitty thing that happened in his life.' Looking back, Meira can see she was so spent from grief that if something Ari did triggered her, she 'wouldn't try, or wouldn't try as hard, to keep my anger in check'. And she had stopped apologising or trying to make amends. 'I think I had this subconscious realisation that because I'm his mother I could get angry at him and he would still love me. I can yell at him and he still comes back and hugs me.' As Meira admitted this, I thought how my children were just the same and I felt a burning mixture of shame, sadness and gratitude.

Neave's birth was not Meira's first experience of birth trauma. She also suffered a massive haemorrhage when Ari was born in 2020. It began when she fell on her stomach while walking down the street at 38 weeks' gestation. She was rushed to hospital, only to spend the next two days waiting, before undergoing an induction. Still, Ari wasn't budging. Then, after more waiting, things suddenly started moving and Meira was pushing. But Ari became stuck and doctors had to deliver him using a vacuum. The placenta should have followed but something went wrong and Meira started bleeding profusely. That time it was she who had to be transferred to a different hospital and she didn't see her son for 24 hours. The massive blood loss and her slow recovery affected their bonding and her breastmilk supply. 'I couldn't even walk to the end of the block for two or three months,' she told me. We talked about how after a traumatic birth, doctors and visitors will often say some version of 'Well, at the end of the day, at least you've got a healthy baby'. 'That's such bullshit, it's such a low bar,' Meira said. 'It made me really angry because it's so unfair, the idea that you completely disappear as soon as your baby is out of your body. I don't think it's fair that it's set up to be like "Well, as long as your baby is healthy, it doesn't matter that you basically die."'

Birth trauma affects one in three Australian women, resulting in physical injuries such as haemorrhaging or tearing, ongoing pain, disability or difficulty going to the toilet or having sex. It can also leave people with psychological trauma if they feared for their life or their baby's life during the birth, if they felt a loss of control, or if their concerns or choices were dismissed or overridden.[1] In 2024, the New South Wales Parliament released a landmark investigation into birth trauma, which stressed that whether a birth experience is traumatic should be decided by the person who goes through it.[2] Some potentially traumatic experiences, like a very long labour or the need for an emergency Caesarean section, may be unavoidable, but the way they happen determines the traumatic impact. A submission to the inquiry by the Centre for Women's Health Research showed those who experienced birth trauma were a staggering 74 per cent more likely to be diagnosed with postnatal depression or anxiety.[3] LGBTQIA+ families, like Meira's, told the inquiry they often had to 'educate' health workers on sexuality, gender and appropriate language.[4] One mother said she was told by a nurse that she would be reported to authorities if she left the hospital when she wanted. She believed she was being penalised as 'a single, gay woman without a second parent for my child'.[5] Another couple were told that the non-birthing spouse would not be allowed to stay in the hospital. And the Aboriginal Health and Medical Research Council explained to the inquiry that many First Nations women find the experience of giving birth in a hospital, away from Country, 'traumatic and frightening' because of a lack of culturally safe care.[6]

For a small group of mothers, a traumatic birth stops them from having more children. The 2023 Australian Birth Experience Study (BESt) by researchers at Western Sydney University surveyed 6100 women who had given birth in the previous five years. One-third said they had experienced a traumatic birth. Among them were 59 women who ruled out a future pregnancy because of their experience, including one whose ordeal in a public hospital 'was so scarring I would never give birth again'. Another 350 mothers said they would not go back to the same hospital, obstetrician or midwife.[7]

After Ari's birth Meira had needed a blood transfusion. Because of this she was scheduled for an extra check-up at four weeks postpartum, in addition to the standard six-week check. She was struggling with breastfeeding and Ari was sleeping for only half an hour at a time during the day and for no more than 90-minute stretches at night. She was still in shock from the birth and spent most of her days walking around like a zombie with her baby strapped to her body. It was also the height of the COVID-19 pandemic and family weren't able to visit from Australia. 'I was so isolated and I was so frightened to talk to or see anyone,' she told me. 'I was really alone all the time.'

At the four-week check a switched-on GP referred her to a psychiatrist. In those early days everything was hard and Meira said she remembers an overwhelming feeling of 'wanting to get my old life back'. Her words slowed as she tried to explain: 'I thought the only way to get back to my old life would be somehow for him to not be there.' She knew she couldn't harm her baby, and she didn't want him to have to live with the knowledge that she'd deserted him by running away. 'So I rationalised that the best thing to do would be for me to, you know [walk] up to the road and then walk into traffic.' She looked at me. 'It wasn't great … so that's when I went on medication, because it was really dark.'

The medication helped with the depression and suicidal thoughts, but it numbed everything else too. 'I didn't get that overwhelming sense of love with Ari for a very long time because I'd had this really traumatic birth and then I had postpartum depression and then I was on antidepressants and mood stabilisers. I liked him, he's really cute, but I was really in the middle [emotionally]. I started to think people were lying about this overwhelming sense of love.'

By the time Ari was about seven months old Meira was starting to feel better – well enough to want to come off the antidepressants. An unexpected side effect was a spike in rage. She found herself having to put her son down in his cot 'so as not to shake him. I would yell at Ari in his crib and be like "Why won't you sleep?" I had no build-up, so I would click into yelling and then click out of it and feel awful.' So Meira resumed the medication for a while. 'The anger was still there sometimes but I was more able to manage it.' Then they lost Neave.

Australian parenting expert Maggie Dent recognises it can be difficult to know how to support a grieving parent, especially as 'everyone responds to the loss of a loved one in their own way'. This can include becoming numb, focusing on others to keep distracted or externalising – 'and mum rage is definitely a part of that', the author, podcast host and mum of four told me when I wrote to ask for her advice. Dent said when women lose their own mother – especially while pregnant or newly postpartum – many tell her they 'feel abandoned and without a rudder'. But we should not underestimate the power of just being there for them, she said. 'Grief can be debilitating as it is exhausting. Allowing mammas to be sad and angry, without trying to cheer them up, is huge.'

Dent, who has worked in palliative care support and conducted more than 200 funerals, gently reminds us not to judge another's grieving process, or ignore or try to minimise their pain. Every parent I've spoken to who has lost a child has echoed this, saying they would prefer that people ask about their child and use their name, rather than pretending nothing has happened because they are nervous to say the wrong thing. For parents who have to explain the death of a family member – including a sibling – to children, Dent urges honesty and simplicity. Give them the facts and answer their questions as best you can, without turning to euphemisms. Creating rituals can also help, like placing a photo in a prominent place in the home and setting aside a spot to display things that remind you of them.

These days, Meira feels she's handling her grief better. She has a regular therapist, although they were hard to find. One told her within a half-hour of meeting her that Meira should sue the hospital. That same therapist also cancelled their second session with 20 minutes' notice, which sparked some rage. Meira is no stranger to therapy. She is married to a trans man and their children are donor-conceived. This meant she had been seeing a therapist during the IVF process. It had taken five cycles to conceive Ari, who grew from one of two embryos frozen on the fifth cycle. Next time around, they used the remaining embryo and Meira fell pregnant with Neave. When she returned to her IVF therapist after Neave died, it quickly became apparent that she wasn't going to be able to help. 'She looked like a deer in the headlights. So I just stopped going.' These days, some of the biggest anger triggers for Meira are seeing other families with a young son and daughter, watching mothers and daughters together, and being confronted with someone else's pregnancy announcement. 'I had this idea of what our family was going to look like,' she said sadly. 'I always said three kids was one too many, but now I would have fifty.'

Part Three

Is This My Life Now?

We are forever changed

After giving birth for the first time, I remember looking at other people with kids and thinking about them in a whole new light. I knew what they'd been through (to an extent). I had a new appreciation for what they were managing behind the scenes. (And, on reflection, I felt a little guilty for not being more helpful to my family and friends who went through it first, when kid-free me had all the time in the world.)

Most of us go into parenting knowing we will have to make sacrifices, and that life will change, but the level of sacrifice and the magnitude of the change are often underestimated. Our life will never be the same. In a survey of Australians conducted over more than two decades, parents – whether they were partnered or single, mums or dads – were asked to rate how much they agreed that parenting was harder than they expected; the average was a score of 4.4 out of a maximum of seven.[1] Indeed, one woman I interviewed for my day job at the newspaper told me new motherhood was harder than anything she'd encountered in her paid work, which happened to involve flying Black Hawk helicopters.

We might not want to fully wind the clock back, but the realisation that we *can't* has the potential to bring about a different kind of grief. We grieve the loss of control and autonomy we had over our lives. We grieve the person we used to be. And that grief can breed resentment, frustration and anger. The problem is that the constant demands of parenting mean we don't have much time to stop and acknowledge that grief for what it is. Or we dismiss it: *I chose to have children and so I chose to give all of that up.* This can be especially complicated for women who have struggled to carry or to adopt their baby, spent considerable financial resources on conceiving, or who have always wanted to be a mum and thought it would be a breeze. Conversely, it can be extra testing for those who may have found themselves unexpectedly or unwillingly thrust into parenthood.

Clinical and counselling psychologist Annabel Hales told me this is common among the women who come to see her. 'It can be grief for the relationships that you used to have before the baby, or changes in your relationship with your partner,' she said. 'You might lose friends or colleagues. You can be grieving identity, grieving changes in your body. Some women might have grief in terms of the sex of that child, they might have wanted a boy or a girl. For some women there is a lot of grief in terms of attention and how that shifts [from them to the baby].' Hales said many mothers don't recognise the grief because we're supposed to be grateful. But if we don't process our grief, she told me, it might come out in the form of resentment. Hales explained that resentment can feel like anger 'but it is more closely aligned with envy ... Women can experience so much envy in motherhood. Envy for our partners who leave the house to go to work, envy for friends who appear to adjust so well and envy for our pre-baby freedom.'

It can be hard to admit that we aren't as selfless in parenthood as we thought we'd be. Our kids are supposed to be our whole world, but giving up the world we knew for them can be a major trigger for mum rage. Parenting means putting someone else first more often than not and forgetting about our own desires for a time. Canadian writer and mother of two Kathryn Jezer-Morton describes this forgetting about ourselves as going into 'camel mode'. In an article for website The Cut in 2023, she explained that when we take on the demands of caring for others we are 'crossing a metaphysical desert of the self without water, like a camel'. In her example, water represents the things you do just for you – the things that bring you joy and spark desire. Camel mode can affect anyone, and last from a few months to years, Jezer-Morton says. We slip into camel mode, often without realising it, because 'it becomes easier – safer – to allow other people's needs to supersede our own'. Camel mode has a kind of numbing effect, helping us to avoid confrontation as we lower our expectations. Getting out takes a concerted effort.[2]

I definitely went into camel mode. (I might still be there …) When I was speaking to a friend who lives overseas, in a rare, snatched phone call when my daughter was less than a year old, she asked what I was up to. Like, other than baby stuff. And I could not think of a single thing I was doing that was not related to our child or our house. In fairness, it was 2020 and a global pandemic was keeping most people indoors. But I had ceased all hobbies. I had no major future plans. Thankfully, this friend has known me since primary school and so I simply confessed to her, 'I'm boring at the moment', confident that she would still be there when I eventually emerged from this phase with more to discuss than which solid food we would be introducing to the baby next. It made sense that at that point in my life I was focused on the shifting sand beneath my feet, not shimmering mirages. But it wasn't until years later that I realised how much the dehydration was affecting my mood.

In the next few chapters, we're going to talk about how the all-encompassing nature of motherhood – and the way it rearranges our lives, bodies and brains – can trigger mum rage. It starts with the actual transition to motherhood, which has been shown to be as brain-altering as puberty,[3] but new mothers are given less slack than grumpy teenagers and less guidance on how it will go or when it will be complete. That first baby arrives, and we're in a blissful bubble. But we have no idea what comes next. After a few weeks or months of groundhog day – wake, feed, change, repeat – we start to realise this is our life now. Then – for many of us – comes the doubt, the overstimulation, the expectations, the loss of identity and the never-ending juggle.

If we thought adolescence (the transition from childhood to adulthood) was stressful, then the transition to motherhood is next level. Like adolescence, it has a name: matrescence. It encompasses the physical, mental and life changes that come with welcoming a child. The term 'matrescence' was coined by anthropologist Dana Raphael. In her 1975 book *Being Female: Reproduction, power, and change* she describes matrescence as 'the time of mother-becoming' and a rite of passage acknowledged differently by different cultures.[4] (Raphael also writes about the significance of patrescence, the transition to fatherhood.)

In recent years, the topic of matrescence has experienced a resurgence as mothers and authors – including Americans Chelsea Conaboy (*Mother Brain*) and Dr Alexandra Sacks (*What No One Tells You*) and Britons Lucy Jones (*Matrescence*) and Zoe Blaskey (*Motherkind*) – have used their platforms to emphasise the power of this word to show mums we're not losing our minds (just reshaping them). As Conaboy put it so beautifully, after bringing a child into the world 'one's organs – brain included – don't simply fit back in place, in their original shape and size and function'.[5] We are forever changed.

Among the growing number of studies that show this is one from 2016 that found notable differences in the brains of women before and after they fell pregnant. The brains of the mums in this study, led by Leiden University in the Netherlands, were also different from other women who did not have children. The changes were so clear that a computer algorithm could pick the mums from the non-mums just by their brain scans.[6] A separate study by the Cognitive Neuroimaging team at Melbourne's Monash University showed the long-lasting effects of matrescence on the brains of Australian women in their late 70s and 80s. It found a relationship between the number of children women had and their memory function.[7]

As I write this book, I am still going through my matrescence. It doesn't finish at your six-week postpartum check-up. It's not over when your baby can walk or your toddler is talking. Or even if you go back to work or have another kid. In the same way adolescence takes years to transform our shape, appearance and brain, matrescence is an ongoing process. When I spoke with *Mom Rage* author and mother of two Minna Dubin, she said she probably didn't emerge from 'the tornado of matrescence' for at least five years after the birth of her first child. 'There are just so many questions that you are trying to figure out,' she said. 'Who am I? How do people see me? How do I see myself?'

All parents struggle in some way as they adjust to their new life. But when it feels like the change is too much to manage, there is a medical term that can be applied. 'Adjustment disorder' is defined as the onset of emotional or behavioural symptoms within three months of a stressor (like, say, having a baby). The symptoms must be either more distressing than one might normally expect in response to the stressful event or they must be impairing a person's ability to function and connect with others as usual.[8]

There are varying opinions on the usefulness of this psychological catch-all phrase, which is applied in major life transitions or periods of uncertainty. Some mothers I spoke to felt it was a 'made-up' thing, or insulting to suggest their struggles were a 'disorder' rather than an understandable reaction to a difficult life phase. 'Just call it matrescence!' one exclaimed. And we definitely should not medicalise every feeling in motherhood as a disorder or condition. But a diagnosis of adjustment disorder allows a GP to refer a patient for further support without necessarily diagnosing postnatal depression or anxiety. PANDA CEO Julie Borninkhof says the term adjustment disorder is 'more palatable' for some mums and adds to our vocabulary to describe the 'diversity of experience'. It has its detractors, but I see adjustment disorder as a gateway for mums who may not think their symptoms are 'bad' or 'textbook' enough to put their hand up for help. It was for me.

Mums and dads aren't necessarily ringing helplines like the one offered by PANDA because of anger or frustration, Borninkhof said, but they're 'worn out emotionally' or in a 'heightened, agitated state'. They feel like they're not reacting to things the way they used to, before kids. Some people are so relieved to have someone to talk to that they spill over with 'everything they've been sitting on or stewing over'. In other cases there are long silences because callers don't have the language to explain how they're feeling. Borninkhof said PANDA staff don't use the word 'rage', which can trouble some parents who are nervous about implying potential risk to their children. But she said they understand the underlying feelings. 'The experience of anger can be one that feels completely out of character and completely overwhelming. We try to normalise the experience of frustration, anger, helplessness or hopelessness.'

Often, just speaking to someone about what's going on and hearing that we're not alone can be enough to stop the meltdown. And we aren't alone. We know mum rage is rife among the Angry Mums Club, and we have learned from the likes of Adrienne Rich and Anne Lamott that mums have been angry for decades. Always, maybe. But is it any worse in the 2020s? Mothering has changed a lot over the decades, influenced by some key people and ideas. As we'll see in the next chapter, they have a bit to answer for when it comes to mum rage.

Mothering ain't what it used to be

Getting angry makes most of us feel like we're a bad mother. But what makes a good mother? It depends on who you ask, and when. Each generation is privy to new science and tools but also weighed down by evolving expectations and norms. University of Melbourne researcher Carla Pascoe Leahy has examined how mothering has evolved since the 1940s, tracing a shift from the 'stoic and pragmatic accounts of postwar mothers to the more personal and expressive' millennial mothers. For her paper 'Maternal metamorphosis: how mothering has changed in Australia since the Second World War', Pascoe Leahy interviewed more than 60 women who became mothers between 1945 and 2022. Each generation had fewer children and spent more time in the workforce. Postwar mums downplayed challenges like breastfeeding and toilet training. In the 1970s and 1980s, access to birth control and sexual education improved and women were more forthcoming about sharing the difficulties of motherhood. From the 1990s onward, motherhood was viewed as a choice rather than a foregone conclusion and women were more focused on establishing careers.[1]

In 2025, a quick scan of the social and mainstream media I'm exposed to paints me a picture of a 'perfect mother' who has all the balls in the air. She cooks the birthday cakes from scratch, her house is clean, she's organised, 'chill' and present – but she also works for pay, has a side hustle or volunteers outside the home. She looks after her health, is fashionable, has at least one hobby, and is up on the latest advice and trends. She never forgets dress-up day or a dentist appointment, she multitasks like a pro, never says no and either hides her burnout or wears it as a badge of honour. She might be tired, but she isn't angry about any of it.

In their book *The Mommy Myth: The idealization of motherhood and how it has undermined all women,* American authors Susan J. Douglas and Meredith W. Michaels lay out in detail the 'enormous role' that television shows, films, magazines, newspapers and social media have 'played in promulgating and exaggerating these myths' about who and what the perfect mother is (at least in Western, white, capitalist society).[2] We are beginning to see more counterpoints to this, especially through social media conversations about #realmotherhood or #motherhoodunplugged. Among the spear carriers for this relatable content are Canadian speaker, author and mum of two Libby Ward (@libbyward) and American podcaster and mum of three Caitlin Murray (@bigtimeadulting), who are both known, and adored, for posting unvarnished videos of themselves, their homes and their parenting struggles and wins. And both have addressed the existence of mum rage head-on. But the perfect mother myth persists. As Douglas and Michaels put it, even if we think the norms of motherhood being beamed at us from every screen are 'preposterous', we still assume we will be 'judged harshly by not abiding by them'.[3]

We are not mothering in a vacuum. We do so in a system of laws, rules, restrictions and expectations. This is what American poet, author and mother Adrienne Rich meant with the subtitle of her book *Of Woman Born*: 'Motherhood as experience and institution'. The obstetricians we see during pregnancy, the experts who write the parenting books, the politicians who pass laws, the bureaucrats who set the rules, the social constructs of marriage and employment – these are all, as Rich describes, 'connecting fibers of this invisible institution'. And, she points out, they influence our relationship with our children 'whether we like to think so or not'.[4]

Australian motherhood studies sociologist Dr Sophie Brock has spent years examining the social conditions and institutions that shape our experiences of being a mother. I talked about her Fish Tank model in an earlier chapter, which illustrates the pressures we face but may not realise we're under. We mums are the fish, confined to a tank (our society) and all its rules and expectations (the water). And depending on where you are in the tank, Dr Brock notes, it can be a lot harder to just keep swimming, as Dory would say. Some fish might be tangled in seaweed or never seem to be able to get to the surface fast enough when the fish flakes are sprinkled.

When I spoke to Dr Brock, I asked what she believed the prevailing definition of a perfect mother was. While it varied across cultures, she said there were some common themes. 'The perfect mother certainly isn't angry. [She] doesn't even have anger as a part of her emotional landscape,' she said. 'She is all-composed, ever-present; she wanted to become a mother. She's fully contented in her role as a mother, she doesn't struggle with feelings like apathy or boredom or anger.' That's the ideal. But, in reality, it is more likely, Dr Brock said, to be a mother who is 'predominantly doing the care work involved in raising children, alone in her house away from extended family ... who experiences relational inequalities in her partnership, who carries the bulk of the domestic load and feels torn between her demands of paid work and parenting'. However, there are also contradictions within the perfect mother myth, Dr Brock warned. If we become mums too young it's no good, but we also shouldn't be too old. We should stay at home to give our kids all our attention, but we should contribute financially to our household somehow (be it selling Tupperware or sponsored social media posts). We should breastfeed, but our baby should also take a bottle when needed. And the rules change over time, and across cultures. Who can keep up?

In researching this book, I read a small library's worth of very good tomes on motherhood. What follows is a short introduction to some of the concepts – and people – who have shaped the way we are mothering today. It is by no means exhaustive. (For a more rigorously academic analysis I highly recommend Nancy Reddy's *The Good Mother Myth*.) One of the names that kept popping up in my reading was sociologist Sharon Hays. In her 1996 book *The Cultural Contradictions of Motherhood* she laid out the central beliefs of what she termed 'intensive mothering' – arguably the most dominant blueprint for how to go about it currently. The rules of intensive mothering tell us children are angelic, they should be cared for primarily by their mother, and the mother's attention, effort and decisions should all revolve around the child's needs. Additionally, intensive mothering is usually 'informed by experts, labor-intensive, and costly'.[5] This means mums should be consulting doctors or tutors, reading all the parenting books and following all the right influencers and experts on social media. They should be playing one-on-one with their children. And they should be buying the best and latest toys or technology, or enrolling their kids in courses and clubs, to further their development. Sound familiar? Hays acknowledges that not every mother will adhere strictly to this model (or have the resources to) but argues that intensive mothering is internalised by most Western parents who will feel some pressure to live up to its ideals. If they don't pass muster there is guilt, and an ever-present feeling that they are responsible for how their children will develop.[6]

The creep of intensive mothering can be seen in how much time we spend with our children. It might feel as if modern-day mothers are busier than ever and spend less quality time with our kids, but data actually says otherwise. A 2005 study by the University of Maryland found modern mothers spend an average of four hours more per week focused on their children than their predecessors in the 1960s. Time diaries of mothers in 1965 found they spent 10.2 hours a week with their children. In 2003 that figure had risen to 14.1 hours. (For comparison, fathers' figures rose from 2.5 to seven hours.) This coincided with a societal focus (verging on paranoia) about child safety, a sharp drop in the time children spent playing on their own, especially away from the house, and a rise in mothers' paid work. While the time mums spent on 'routine' care like feeding and bathing remained steady, time spent on 'interactive' activities like reading or playing with children spiked. (That would be intensive mothering in action ...) Interestingly, all this reduced the time mums spent on housework, cooking and cleaning by more than 13 hours per week between 1965 and 2000.[7]

Another study, by academics at the University of California, Irvine, found the amount of time parents spent with their children rose between 1965 and 2012 in all but one of 11 Western nations. (French mothers were the exception.) The time mothers spent doing things like feeding, bathing and dressing children, reading, playing or helping with homework almost doubled from an average of 54 minutes a day in 1965 to 104 minutes in 2012. In comparison, fathers' time with their kids nearly quadrupled – from a 'scant' base of just 16 minutes to 59 minutes.[8]

The pressures of intensive mothering apply to both stay-at-home mums and those who work for pay but, infuriatingly, its key requirements are in direct conflict with the expectations of workers in a capitalist society. As Hays explains, the ideal worker is meant to strive for individual success, productivity and profit – the opposite of putting someone else first all the time and expending a lot of money doing it. Hays says the pervasive influence of intensive mothering ideals means mums have little genuine choice about whether they adhere. Their 'choice' is whether to add paid work to the mix. This scenario sets up a false and unhelpful division between stay-at-home mums and so-called 'supermums', dubbed the 'mommy wars'. This term was launched into the popular vernacular by

Newsweek journalist Nina Darnton in a 1990 article titled 'Mommy vs. mommy'. The piece pitted the motivations and efforts of stay-at-home mothers against those who worked for pay. Using battle terms like 'opening salvo' and 'direct hit', Darnton described how these two types of mums trade barbs and fire passive–aggressive insults in the fight to prove who is doing best by their children.[9] But, as Douglas and Michaels remind us in *The Mommy Myth*, most mums actually come and go from the workforce at certain stages, rather than adhering to 'ironclad' roles on one or other side.[10]

Before intensive mothering there was attachment parenting, which is pretty intense too. And really, it should be called 'attachment mothering' because it's largely about having the child physically attached to mum. The approach was promoted by Dr William (Bill) Sears and his wife Martha Sears in wildly popular *The Baby Book*, first published in 1992. The hallmarks of attachment parenting are breastfeeding (ideally for as long as the child wants), co-sleeping with infants in your bed or in a bassinet right next to it, and baby-wearing in a sling or carrier. Letting a baby cry for long without attention is a big no-no. I'd not heard of *The Baby Book* when I became a mum but it turns out I followed every one of these tenets in some way. I thought I was doing these things for my own reasons. I breastfed because I was able (although it is also very strongly encouraged in Australian birthing hospitals and I got the impression that if I could, I should). Our babies slept in a bassinet next to my bed for months and I sometimes co-slept when they were older, out of sheer desperation to get some shut-eye. And I got a lot of use out of our clip-on baby carrier, especially when our second child came along, because it freed my hands. I didn't do these things because I feared that *not* doing them would somehow damage my kids (at least not consciously). But it seems some mothers do.

Part of the problem is that attachment parenting sounds a lot like attachment theory, a separate concept that evolved largely from the work of British psychoanalyst John Bowlby and American-Canadian developmental psychologist Mary Ainsworth in the 1950s. The theory goes that children need a relationship with a primary carer (usually mum) that provides a 'secure base' from which they can venture out and come back safely.[11] Securely attached infants, it is argued, are more likely to have better outcomes later in life (although the theory faces criticism for focusing too narrowly on the biological mother being the only truly acceptable secure base).

As *TIME* magazine journalist Kate Pickert explained in a deep dive into attachment parenting and the Searses in 2012, in an article headlined 'The man who remade motherhood', the theory and the parenting style are often confused. Mums end up thinking that if they don't strictly follow the rules of attachment parenting then their kid will end up with insecure attachment. But, as Pickert points out, attachment theory developed from the study of children orphaned or abandoned by their mothers, not 'well-parented children who are fed formula (instead of breast milk) and put in bouncy seats (instead of slings)'.[12]

The central pillars of attachment parenting touch on some of the most emotional, contentious and divisive aspects of mothering (and the anxiety and guilt they can conjure). If we have working mum versus stay-at-home mum in the 'mommy wars', then we also have breastfeeding mum versus bottle-feeding mum, sleep-training mum versus sleep-with-the-kid-in-my-bed-every-night mum, and pick-my-kid-up mum versus let-them-cry-it-out mum. Of course, these aren't really 'types' of mums. And none of these choices is right or wrong. But that's the whole point. No matter which parenting 'style' we try to adhere to, we can feel like we're not living up to its standards.

On the heels of the attachment and intensive models of mothering, we now have the expectation that we will all engage in 'gentle parenting'. The hallmark move of the gentle parent is to get down to eye level with our kid, say, just after they've hit their sister or thrown spaghetti all over the white walls, and ask about their feelings. We must keep our cool in the process, modelling emotional regulation. And don't even think about introducing any punishments (or even rewards) into the equation. Gently parented kids are meant to follow our example to develop an inner moral compass unaffected by sticker charts or threats that Santa won't visit this year. Or as journalist, author and mum Jessica Winter wrote in *The New Yorker* in 2022: the child becomes a person who is 'self-regulating, kind, and conscientious because she wants to be, not because it will result in ice cream'.[13] (Oops, too late ...)

In the 2020s, there has been an explosion of gentle parenting content on social media, offering us step-by-step scripts to use with children to understand what their behaviour is really signalling. Like so many parents of my generation, I am acutely aware of this style of interacting with our children – and feel pressure to follow it so I don't otherwise totally mess up my kids. When I have the bandwidth, I have named feelings with an agitated toddler and sat calmly through a preschooler's meltdown. I have told my children, 'I'm here' and 'I get it'. Sometimes it helps de-escalate tantrums and I do think the language seeps into their vocabulary, which will hopefully add to their emotional intelligence in adulthood. But it can be exhausting, and unrealistic. A 2022 paper titled 'The cult of the child' explained how this era of parenting 'places the interests of children above all others' and leans towards an 'exclusively positive' approach, which explicitly rules out the use of punishment, discipline, 'timeouts and intentional ignoring'.[14] Hands up if you've tried any of those? In my interviews with parents in their 30s, most of them aspired to gentle parenting, often because they feared they would be scarring their children emotionally if they yelled or disciplined like their parents did. But this pressure to always be calm and gentle is creating another trigger for mum rage, especially if we feel we've failed to get it right.

Genevieve, a cusp millennial mum in her late 30s like me, agrees that our generation of parents feels a heavy burden to get the emotional aspects of parenting spot on. We're all starting to understand how much our childhoods shaped us and 'expectations are so much higher on us with that knowledge'. Genevieve and her husband 'subscribe to a form of gentle parenting as much as possible', she told me as we waited in line to grab takeaway lunch during her break from work in Adelaide's CBD. They try to reason with their four-year-old and 'let him express his emotions and normalise when he's upset', even though she acknowledges this is probably not the way she was raised. 'My parents may have done a bit of that but certainly they were way more disciplinary and authoritarian,' she said. 'And we laugh about it now because, with the grandkids, they're massive softies and the biggest walkovers.' But even those who aspire to gentle parenting can find themselves wanting to abandon a tantrumming kid (or at least lock themselves in the bathroom for five minutes when it all gets too much). 'It's those tiny things that add up and eventually it escalates when they really push you over the edge,' Genevieve said. 'And what if we're in public? What am I going to do, leave him in the supermarket? He has all the bargaining power there. I just want to get my loaf of bread and my tampons and get home.'

Paediatric psychologist Terence Sheppard believes this perceived difficulty involved in parenting today is a driving factor in many young women choosing to put off having kids. 'It feels all too hard,' he told me during an interview for *The Advertiser*'s *SA Weekend* magazine at his suburban clinic in Adelaide, 'but we are making it too hard. We are overcomplicating the task of parenting and we are overdoing the amount of energy it really requires.' Dr Sheppard and his paediatrician wife Dr Margaret Kummerow have raised three children to adulthood and spent their careers working with kids. In 2024 they released *Positive Parenting: A guide to raising psychologically healthy children*, a book which urges us to dial back the intensity. Allow our children to be bored for a moment (including in – shock horror – timeout). Send them off to play on their own or figure something out for themselves. Make them wait their turn rather than interrupting your conversation or your toilet break. Dr Sheppard says much of the pressure parents feel stems from a fear that 'people will think I'm a bad mother, or a bad parent, if I don't attend to my child. That a good mother or a good father will drop everything at a moment's notice in order to resolve a child's needs.'

Clinical psychologist Nicole Williams sees this pressure internalised by many of the women who come to see her after having kids. 'There is this binary between good mother and bad mother, and being angry and being calm, but that is really unhelpful,' she told me. 'In this context a "good mother" is essentially happy and joyful and grateful ... but no one is all that, all the time. We can feel those things but also we're hungry and we're bored and we're tired and we're ambivalent and we're angry.'

Dr Williams stresses the importance of *feeling* our feelings in front of our kids, as long as we're prepared to do the necessary follow-up. 'I get angry at my kids,' she said. 'I will raise my voice at times and I will not necessarily feel amazing about that, but I'll come back and I'll repair the hell out of that. They learn amazing things from having those experiences of someone being able to come back and say, "That wasn't really how I want to behave, that mustn't have been very nice for you, and here's what I'm going to try to do about it."'

Two-thirds of Angry Mums Club members said that they apologised to their kids after an outburst and about the same number tried to explain their feelings to their child. A quarter said they tried to justify the outburst to themselves or others, while 10 per cent blamed it on someone else's actions (like their kid or partner). Only 3 per cent moved on as if nothing had happened.

Dr Williams wants her clients to know that the difference between her and them is not that she doesn't get angry. 'It's that I don't beat myself up about the fact that I get angry. I can close the door and leave it, and it doesn't add to my volcano erupting.'

While the societal pressure to be an intensive, attached, gentle parent remains strong, there are some mums bucking the trend, like my News Corp colleague Dr Susie O'Brien, author of *The Secret of Half-arsed Parenting*.[15] Her method is the opposite of intensive; a just-enough-to-get-by approach that saves time and energy for the things that really keep a family together. We share the attitude that jettisoning the low-hanging fruit and giving up on other people's expectations makes parenting easier (and therefore less rage-inducing). It was in Dr O'Brien's book that I learned about author and podcaster Holly Wainwright's 'I Don't' list. Published by Mamamia in 2019, Wainwright's viral list included admissions like 'I don't iron', 'I don't make birthday cakes' and 'I don't meal prep'. And most importantly, she doesn't feel guilty about not doing things she used to think she should.[16] (Axe the guilt, remember, and actively resist others' expectations.) Wainwright's confessions prompted an avalanche of reciprocal unloading from mums around Australia who don't change the sheets every week, exercise every day or have a tidy house. After reflecting on the triggers for my mum rage, and trying to claw back some time and energy for the things that matter, I don't dust shelves, strive to make Insta-worthy school lunches or feel guilty when I use the clothes dryer. And I do not put the elf on the shelf. What could you outsource, automate or scrap altogether?

This idea of not having to be perfect can actually be interpreted in the instructions of a man who shaped how millions of mothers viewed their role in the middle of last century. English paediatrician and psychoanalyst Donald Winnicott first spoke to women across Britain through wartime BBC broadcasts in the 1940s, assuring them that motherhood was the role they were born to play and doing it well would come naturally if they just followed their instincts.[17] In his now widely quoted model of the 'good enough mother', Winnicott says a new mum will start out attending to every squawk of her infant, in 'almost complete adaptation' to the baby's needs. At first this near-obsession is necessary, being that infant humans are completely reliant on others for their survival. But over time the good enough mother gradually and deliberately starts to pull back, adapting less and less in line with her baby's 'growing ability to deal with her failure'.[18] Except failure here is actually what the baby needs so that they can begin to develop some autonomy. Let's be clear though: for Winnicott this freeing up of the mother had nothing to do with what she might need or want, how she might spend that spare time and energy. It was entirely in service of the baby. Winnicott may not have necessarily meant his theory to be a comfort to women that they didn't have to be perfect. But there's no reason why we can't interpret his instructions as permission to ease up on perfection, knowing our kid will be ok. It might even be good for them.

One particular study shows us just how often most of us are missing the mark in mothering – and that it isn't the end of the world. In 1989, American developmental psychologist Edward Tronick and his colleague Jeffrey Cohn examined face-to-face interactions between 54 pairs of mothers and babies aged between three and nine months to see how coordinated or in sync they were. Their study found mum and baby were 'mismatched' or trying to get back in sync more than 70 per cent of the time. In other words, they were getting it wrong far more often than they were getting it right. The authors concluded that it was 'common', 'expected' and 'normal' for mums and bubs to be on different pages.[19] The important part, as Dr Williams also told us, was the time they spent in a 'process of repair' to fix the misunderstanding.

The first time I went to see a psychologist about my mum rage, she raised the 'good enough' concept with me. She essentially suggested that we're all frustrated by our kids and if I was working to repair with mine when things got out of hand, then I shouldn't be so hard on myself. I remember initially thinking something like: *Why did I bother to see a professional if you're just going to give me that 'you're doing a great job' line?* But the more I thought about it, I realised that hearing this from a woman who saw many people with many problems, many of them mothers, was validating. She was telling me I wasn't alone. She was telling me I wasn't bad for getting mad. She was telling me mothering feels hard because it *is* hard and I should cut myself some slack.

Relentless provocation

For as long as I can remember, I knew I wanted kids. I longed for the day I would hear someone call me 'Mum'. When our daughter began babbling 'mumumum', it was the best thing I'd ever heard. I can recall the exact morning I heard her call out 'Mummy' for the first time, as I watched her in her cot on the baby monitor. What I didn't know was just how many times I would hear that word, or some variation of it, every day of my life thereafter! It still makes my stomach flip when I come through our front door and my kids run to me yelling, 'Mummy, Mummy, Mummy'. But there's also the barrage of requests fired from the back seat of the car, or the constant calling out from the toilet, their bed, the backyard or the other room. 'Mum, look at this.' 'Mum, can I have that?' 'Mum, where are you?' 'Mum, I'm hungry.' One day, after fielding a blast of 'Mums' in quick succession, I wondered how many times a day I hear, and have to respond or choose not to respond to, that word. So, in June 2024, when my kids were two and four, I decided to find out. I bought a traffic click counter, one of those ones with a lever you press with your thumb each time you want to increase the count, and began my experiment.

The first time I used it was on a Saturday and I was home on my own with the kids while their dad was out for the day.

I didn't remember to start using the clicker until 7 am. By 9 am I had clicked that thing 173 times. That's more than once every minute. By 11 am the rate had slowed considerably, totalling 230, as I'd abandoned our four walls for the distraction of an indoor play café. (More running, less 'Mum'ing.) By bedtime, 12 hours after the first click, the number on the counter was 421. That's an average of at least one 'Mum' every two minutes. All. Day. Long. And here's the thing: I didn't realise until I started this experiment how good I had become at tuning out some of the 'Mums', so I am positive this is an underestimate.

Circumstances can change the count dramatically. I kept clicking for the next fortnight and the mum count varied greatly depending on how much time I spent with the kids. The next morning, a Sunday, I am not lying when I tell you I counted 118 Mums from my daughter before she even got out of bed. I'd put the clicker on my nightstand when I went to sleep the night before and when I heard her call out just before 6 am I started pressing. Usually, I'd get up and go to her but, just to see what happened, I lay there as the count rose. 'Mum. Mum. Mummy. Mamaaaa. Mummyyyyy. Muuuuuum.' Eventually, I threw off the covers and kept clicking as I wandered down the hallway to her room.

By the end of the day, with their father at home, the total Mum count was about halved, showing 250 by 6.20 pm. That was also when my son grabbed the device off the kitchen bench and started madly clicking away, ruining any chance of further data collection. (For those asking at this juncture 'What about the dads?' I didn't count the D-word because if I were around to do so my kids would still be saying Mum. Perhaps I could have hidden in the laundry or something, but that would have been a waste of alone time.) On Monday, I counted 94 Mums by 9 am, at which point I dropped our eldest off to kindy and the Mum count slowed with half the children present. We hit 264 by bedtime that night. On Tuesday we clocked 163 Mums between 6 am and 9 am. The kids were at kindy and childcare for most of the day, but there was a late flurry as they burst through the front door that evening, bringing the day's total Mum count to 252. The rest of the week both my partner and I worked full days and the kids were in childcare so the count dropped to between 83 and 143 Mums per day. The lowest tally recorded over the fortnight was 55, on a childcare day when they slept in (and I likely stuck them in front of the TV at some point). Aside from the record 421 on the first day, I also fielded a respectable 387 Mums the following Sunday. For context, a year after my experiment, another Australian mum, Jasmine, went viral for conducting her own Mum count with the same nifty clicker. In a TikTok video she counted the number of Mums said by her four-year-old daughter and two-year-old son. She started at 7 am. By 8 pm her count reached 234.[1]

That's a lot of numbers for someone who does words for a living, but I include these figures to drive home the point that mothers are constantly called on to listen, assess, respond and redirect. (Remember Dolf Zillmann's 'sequence of provocations'?) If my click counter data isn't the epitome of overstimulation, I don't know what is. Among the Angry Mums Club 53 per cent identified overstimulation as a trigger for melting down. This put it second on the list of factors that most contributed in the moment of an outburst, behind a child not listening. When asked what played into their anger in motherhood over time, not just at the moment of explosion, 55 per cent identified the relentlessness of parenting. They used words like 'exhausted', 'tapped out', 'touched out' and 'overwhelmed'. They told of early wake-ups – every day – no holidays, no sick leave, endless loads of washing and dinner every damn night. And the questions! The constant questions. An average of 288 of them a day, in fact.

That figure comes from a survey of 1000 British mothers of children aged between two and ten, conducted by retailer Littlewoods. It found, on average, that kids in that age bracket ask 288 questions between 7.19 am and 7.59 pm each day. Nine-year-old boys ask the least questions, at *just* 144. And the most? Four-year-old girls are firing 390 queries at us in a 12-and-a-half-hour period.[2] That's more than one question every two minutes, from the time they wake to the time they (finally) shut their eyes after reading three books, having a drink of water, taking a trip to the toilet and listening to two chapters of a *Winnie the Pooh* audiobook played through the Bluetooth-connected speaker in their room. That might sound like an oddly specific description but all I can say is, as I write this chapter, I am living with a particularly chatty four-year-old girl.

It's probably karma, as I was a really talkative kid. And as someone who now gets paid to ask questions for a living, I don't want to discourage her curiosity. But there is arguably a bit of a difference between 'Minister, why were you not told about the girl who fell pregnant while under your watch in state care?' and 'Mum, did you know that Mayor Goodway in *Paw Patrol* has a pet chicken?' And the timing counts too. Most mornings I have fielded three or four questions before I've properly opened my eyes or emptied my bladder. Sometimes an insightful query will catch me by surprise, like 'Why do trains have different wheels to buses?' Then there are mortifying ones like 'Mum, how old are you? Are you 87?' and the plain adorable ones like 'When I'm a parent can I eat as much chocolate as I want too?'

In recent years there's been a trend in social media content riffing off the theme 'Mums aren't angry, we're just overstimulated'. The kinds of questions coming from my kids every day, and my click count, show just how stimulating an environment we're in. As we've already covered, there are plenty of legitimate reasons why mums get angry. Feeling overstimulated might be the thing that causes us to snap, but by now we know that we are usually that close to a meltdown because of other underlying factors. On a day when we've had too little sleep and we're trying to juggle paid work and 390 questions from a preschooler on an empty stomach, we are much more likely to be pushed off the edge by overstimulation than if we are well rested, with a manageable to-do list and a moment to ourselves. It's about giving our higher-order brain bits at least a fighting chance of being able to step in and save us from ourselves (or our amygdalae).

Kylie, the stay-at-home mum who lives in country New South Wales, told me a relatable story of her struggle to juggle too many competing demands. At the time she wrote to me she had a two-year-old son and a six-month-old daughter. They had returned home from grocery shopping and Kylie desperately needed to wee. She laid her daughter on the floor outside the bathroom, in her line of sight, with some toys. 'I knew she was tired, and she started hysterically crying, but I couldn't wait to go to the bathroom,' the 27-year-old explained. (There's our brain's salience network doing its thing.) As Kylie rushed for the loo, her son followed. With a backing soundtrack of her daughter's wails, her son began unravelling the toilet paper, tearing tiny bits off and dropping them all over the floor. Already on the throne by this point, Kylie told him to stop. Then she tried to distract him by suggesting he go and get a toy for his sister, but he wasn't interested. 'All the while my daughter is screaming and there's more and more mess piling up,' Kylie recounted. 'Then I just can't hold it [the anger] in anymore. I feel it in my chest. I grab my son's hand and scream, "Hey, I said stop that" at a volume that was unnecessary and shameful.' Kylie said this was a classic example of how 'having competing noise and tasks really triggers me'.

Another time she was trying to change her baby's nappy, with her toddler pulling at her leg and her husband talking to her from the other end of the room. Then her baby put a wayward foot in the pooey nappy and Kylie snapped. 'I yelled something like, "Stop moving," and then stomped my feet and did a weird little closed-mouthed scream.' In moments like this Kylie said, the rage 'comes over me so quickly and so unexpectedly and I feel out of control … Once I have an outburst, I feel like I need to literally stomp my feet or throw something or act out like a child. I just feel it so physically. I feel so much guilt and shame about it afterwards but I cannot control it.'

For Kylie, the rage started after the birth of her second child, who had 'a vastly different temperament that I was wildly unprepared for'. In hindsight, she and her husband call their son their 'false confidence baby'. 'He slept every night, never cried, ate food easily,' she told me. 'I felt like wonder mum.' But his sister 'entered the world screaming' and kept it up for the next four months. 'She didn't sleep, she wanted to breastfeed constantly, she wanted to be held all the time. She had reflux and nappy rash and every bug and cold her brother brought home from childcare.' When I asked Kylie whether she ever expected to feel angry as a mum she told me she 'knew to look out for, and even expect, depression, but rage was just never on my radar. I thought I'd be an "I'm not mad, I'm just disappointed" kind of parent, not a "lose my temper over the smallest thing" kind of parent.' (Same …)

Kylie's struggle is compounded by the fact that her husband doesn't get it. He's 'hands-on' with the kids, she said, and they agree on most of the parenting basics, but he can't comprehend her rage. 'I often take a lot of anger out on him when he gets home from work because he doesn't understand the urgency I feel when I say I need something from him. But I feel like when I'm angry with my husband it's for a reason. With the kids, it feels like it comes out of nowhere.' One day, after Kylie confided in her husband about the intensity of her feelings, he told her she didn't seem like the person he married anymore. 'That filled me with shame,' she said.

For a growing number of women, the transition to motherhood and the overstimulation that comes with it is leading to a diagnosis of attention deficit hyperactivity disorder in adulthood. To be clear, ADHD is a neurological condition a person is born with, and has been dealing with since childhood – even if they didn't realise. There has been a surge in adult diagnoses post-pandemic, particularly among women, and this has drawn criticism that many are jumping on the bandwagon of a 'trend'. But there is a burgeoning conversation around how the hormonal upheaval of pregnancy or the massive increase in executive functioning capacity required to look after more people in a household can bring to light ADHD symptoms that might have previously been managed, masked or misunderstood. The extra time demands of parenting also strip most of us of the time we used to have to engage in coping strategies like regular exercise, sleep and meals or alone time to decompress. Quite often parents are being diagnosed after recognising themselves in the process of getting a child assessed for the condition. When British journalist and author Grace Timothy was diagnosed her daughter was eight years old. Timothy shares in her 2025 book *Is It My ADHD?* how the diagnosis helped her understand why things like noise, conflict and the spike in life admin that comes as children reach school age exacerbated her frustration in motherhood. '[I] find it hard to shake the default of shouting when I feel challenged,' she wrote. 'I know what kind of mother I want to be; less shouty ... but it's never as easy or as natural as I thought.'[3]

ADHD Australia describes the condition as a complex neuro-developmental disorder characterised by 'persistent patterns of inattentive, impulsive, and sometimes hyperactive behaviour', which are 'frequently accompanied by emotional regulation challenges'. The organisation estimates one in 20 Australian adults have the condition.[4] A number of women in the Angry Mums Club named neurodivergence as a factor contributing to their difficulties in managing their emotions in motherhood. One said that being diagnosed with ADHD and starting medication had 'changed absolutely everything ... I don't have anywhere near the amount of rage and overload

I used to. I just wish I had been medicated sooner so I could have avoided being so awful,' she wrote.

Meira, who we met earlier, was diagnosed at the age of 36, after the birth of her first child, Ari. In hindsight, she wonders why it took that long. 'I look back now and it was clear that I had really strong emotional dysregulation. I definitely was an angry kid and an angry teenager,' the now 39-year-old reflected. Meira said she developed coping strategies and regular routines in her 20s, but then she had a baby and 'you drop all your balls. I have no runway, I go from snapping to rage,' she explained. 'I can't have caffeine or I'm flying off the walls. And I really need routines ... and time on my own.'

For Laura, getting her ADHD diagnosis at 44 was bittersweet. Before that she just thought she was 'a shit parent' who 'wasn't coping'. Laura describes overload as a common trigger for her mum rage. 'That's what trips the switch, that one thing when you've got that many things already in your hands and your brain. It feels like a pile of rocks just falling down on me and then that breaking point. That's what makes me snap.' Before raising her girls with her husband, Laura had systems to help her organise and remember things. 'When kids came into my life I would try to keep the systems, but they move things or change things and then everything goes out the window.' Now that she has been diagnosed and is taking medication she said she wants to go back and do those years parenting her littlies again. 'I still get the overload but it's different now. If something goes bad in the morning I can take it in my stride. Before, it would have thrown me out and it would be like an explosion. The guilt I have about that is like nothing I've ever felt.'

More kids = more anger?

When my son was about nine months old, I found myself in one of those shopping centre parent rooms. You know, the ones with the nappy change tables and the toddler toilet next to the adult-sized one. On entering, it took me a moment to register that the five kids in front of me – ranging in age from what I guessed was about 12 down to a newborn – all appeared to belong to one woman. Then I noticed there was a sixth child in the closed toilet cubicle. The presumed mother seemed calm and in control. When the kid in the cubicle was done she gathered the brood and they filed out, leaving me gawping in their wake. I was surprised, impressed and a bit jealous.

I would have liked to have tried for more children, but my partner was quite happy to have a girl and a boy, and not keen to return to the newborn phase. I must admit I felt some shame about this because part of the reason he didn't want to go there again is that it was so emotionally tumultuous for our household. It turns out I'm not the only one to have grappled with this. In *The Good Mother Myth*, American academic and mum of two Nancy Reddy shares how she feared her husband might veto a second baby because of her 'dark fury' and 'frustration which, at any moment, could spring open from the locked box of my heart' in those difficult, early days of parenting.[1] In time, I have come to feel fulfilled by our family just the way it is, but I think often about what it would be like to be a mum of many.

According to the Australian Institute of Family Studies, in the early 1980s about one-third of Australian mothers in their mid-to-late 40s had four or more children. By 2016 that proportion had dropped to 11 per cent. In contrast, the proportion of mothers who have one child almost doubled from about 8 per cent in 1981 to 14 per cent in 2016.[2] These days, two kids are most common – for myriad reasons in or out of parents' control. People are leaving baby-making until later (by choice, or not) and the ever-rising cost of living can make big-family budgeting a daunting prospect. But those mega families are out there. During my second pregnancy I joined an online group where women from around Australia were posting about having their eighth, tenth or even – in one case – twelfth child. Blog posts by mums of that many kids often lament the 'gawk' factor, where people stare at siblings piling out of a mini-van or ask offensive questions like whether the parents 'meant' to have that many. Queensland's Bonell family is believed to be one of Australia's largest. Mum Jeni and dad Ray have 16 children aged from seven to their mid-30s. Their nine sons and seven daughters are all biological offspring with no multiple births. From the age of eight the Bonell children join the family jobs roster, helping to cook and clean (how's that for automation?!). In an interview published by Mamamia, Jeni said while it was incredibly (but unsurprisingly) difficult to get time alone, the 'joys' of a large family outweighed the negatives. She did also note it takes 'a bucket load of tolerance to handle so many children'.[3] (I bet …)

It was harder than I expected to get mums of many to talk to me for this book. One I approached specifically told me mum rage is not something she struggles with. A few others were probably just too busy to get back to me. But I did speak to Giulia Jones, the mum of six in Canberra, and Shona Reid, a mum of seven in Adelaide. In surprising news to me, both women dismissed the suggestion that more kids mean more anger. Instead, they argued, it means more experience and more hands to help. 'You're fully busy with two and it doesn't really get much worse after that,' said Jones, whose six children range in age from six to 18. 'I only felt truly overwhelmed with my sixth child. I was unwell with my sixth baby and ended up with a hysterectomy, so there was going to be no more babies anyway.'

Jones said having a role model who managed a large brood helped. 'My mum handled five kids so I already knew it could be done. Mothers of big families have got into a rhythm and they've really been able to test what they can handle. They know to drop trying to be some things that they can't be, and to drop getting worked up about every single thing. It doesn't really matter if the kids' room is covered in toys. You just learn to shut a door and not look. And you learn the sounds that are "something I need to respond to" versus "something I don't need to respond to". That is a very finely tuned skill,' she said, with a laugh.

Reid is a proud Eastern Arrernte mother of seven children, ranging in age from nine to 31. And then there's her brother's children, and her cousins' kids. 'They all call each other brothers and sisters so our families are huge,' Reid said. She and other Aboriginal mums I spoke to felt there was a safety in large sibling groups because the older children looked out for the young ones, settling babies, holding bottles, and entertaining and looking out for each other. 'It's almost like I've relinquished part of my sense of control because there's another person in their world who's got their back, who loves them and cares for them. So I can sit in the knowledge that that's okay.'

But what if you get two – or more – kids at once? Among the Angry Mums Club one mother told me her rage was triggered when she had twins and she transformed into a mum of three overnight. Another recalled her anger escalating after baby number two and 'significantly' worsening after number three came along – all before the eldest turned five.

In Adelaide, Elke's first and only pregnancy brought her and husband Alex identical twin girls. 'I expected to be tired and for it to be hard work, but I was completely unprepared for the total lack of control, the frustration and the fury of being plunged into the chaos of constantly crying or whinging children,' Elke, 40, told me. The girls were born prematurely and spent their first month in the special care nursery. Elke caught public transport every day (because she couldn't drive after a C-section) to breastfeed her twins, which she continued for 15 months. When the couple brought their babies home the teeny pair 'screamed relentlessly' – in the car, in the pram, in the house. They rarely slept at the same time and it felt like too much to ask family or friends to look after not one but two babies. 'There was … no promise of a break or someone taking them off my hands,' Elke said. 'For so long my husband did not feel comfortable taking them on his own so I had to be around them all the time. I was constantly frustrated. I so badly wanted to love them and nurture them but they took everything from me.'

The twins are now 'bright, helpful, capable' preteens. But those rage-inducing early years are seared in Elke's memory. Once while sitting between two bassinets, patting a child on either side in a desperate bid to get them to sleep simultaneously, she found herself 'patting a bit harder and then I just screamed. I absolutely screamed at the top of my lungs for them to "*Shut up!*" I slammed the door and just left them.' Another time Elke was trying to get shoes on one of her daughters, who was by then a toddler and was resisting and whining. It came after a long stint of this behaviour and Elke had reached her limit. 'I just pushed her off my lap and screamed at her, [asking] why did she have to make everything so difficult?' Elke's other daughter witnessed the outburst and looked at Elke, 'terrified'.

Elke and Alex sought help from Torrens House, a government-funded unit in Adelaide for parents with babies under 12 months who are struggling with feeding, settling or sleeping. They rang the nurses and social workers at the Parent Helpline, and sought the support of the national Multiple Births Association community. But Elke says the 'traumatic rollercoaster of fury' she experienced in the early years has forever changed her. 'I want to scream at the top of my lungs about helping parents of multiples so much more.'

Extra kids might bring extra triggers in some households, while in others they can form a well-oiled machine that takes some weight off mum's shoulders. A troupe of busy siblings might never be home while an only child's emotional or behavioural needs may be all-encompassing for their one-and-done parents. Quite often the kids are actually the least of our worries. We love them and want to spend *more* quality time with them. It's all the other shit – the constant housework, the paid work, the planning, negotiating and bettering ourselves – that gets us steaming. It's time to look at how the environment we're mothering in, and the one we grew up in, land some of us straight in a pressure cooker rather than a cold pot on the stove.

Part Four

It Feels Hard Because It Is

The self-care squeeze

Imagine, for a moment, that this is your life. You wake after a terrible night's sleep, interrupted not only by your children but also by motorcyclists doing burnouts on the nearby main road, a police helicopter hovering overhead, sirens in the streets or loud neighbours partying. Throwing off the blankets, you're hit by a shock of cold air because the heater is broken, or too expensive to run. You've got to scrape together breakfast and get the kids dressed and packed. You don't have a car, or you're low on petrol, so you have to take the bus. It's a mission to keep the kids under control on public transport and you can feel the judging eyes of other passengers as they squabble loudly with each other. After you finally get the older ones to school you have to do a supermarket trip with the baby, and you don't have enough cash to buy all the things you need, let alone want.

Back home, after getting the baby down for a nap, you apply for jobs but there aren't many with hours you could feasibly work. There's time for a rushed tidy up around the house, and then it's back to school to pick up hungry, tired kids and get them all fed, washed and into bed. Through it all, you've been ignoring a niggling pain in your hip that you can't attend to because there's no bulk-billing GP close enough to home, or you keep forgetting to call about the appointment. You know your mental health is sliding but there's no way you can afford the psychologist gap fee, or find the time to see one, so why bother. And this happens on repeat, every day. So when you wake up the next morning to do it all over again, your stress threshold is already near breaking point. All it takes is the baby waking just after your eyelids have closed, your five-year-old refusing to put on their shoes or the tweenager sulking about not having the latest something or other and you snap. Maybe you don't even need to *imagine* this scenario. This is everyday life, or something like it, for many mums. It is Zillmann's 'sequence of provocations' on repeat.

Experienced social worker Sally Rhodes says mums in these situations are often not aware of how close to the edge they are until they go over it. 'They're always in a state of hyper arousal and it doesn't take much to tip them into fear, and then terror,' says Rhodes, who founded Connecting Families SA. 'They're not regulated. You can't be regulated when you're in that state. And they're in that state most of the time.'

These effects can be seen on brain scans. American developmental neuroscientist Pilyoung Kim and colleagues scanned the brains of 53 first-time mums within ten months of giving birth. All were on low or middle incomes and experiencing varied levels of stressful circumstances like food insecurity, poor housing, community violence or financial shortfalls. During the scans they were asked to listen to the sound of a baby crying. The researchers found that the more stressed mothers were not as sensitive to the sound, and had reduced activity in parts of the brain involved in parenting, including prioritising, evaluating emotional cues, processing emotional information and regulating emotions.[1] Another US study of almost 300 low-income mums found that not being able to buy enough nappies to change infants when needed was more stressful to mothers than not being able to afford enough food.[2]

The socioeconomic status of parents does not automatically determine their ability to cope, or mean they are any more likely to be neglectful or violent. But research has found that they might be more likely to develop burnout. A 2022 study involving about 3400 mostly Belgian, French and Swiss adults – half of whom were from low socioeconomic backgrounds – found that when parents are in survival mode it can be hard to focus on the needs of their children. In such cases, neglect isn't a conscious choice so much as 'the consequence of exhaustion' from the challenges of their life.[3]

So if we think about that fictional mum at the beginning of this chapter, when does she get time to try to turn down the heat before she melts down? How does she squeeze even a moment of self-care into her daily grind? Self-care means different things to different mums. Taking a bath or getting a pedicure for some, going for a run, reading a book or sleeping in for others. It could also be organising a night out with friends or even saying yes to a solo interstate work opportunity (when you'll get some time to yourself on the aeroplane). Equally, it can be going to bed early. Eating a vegetable when you'd rather a chocolate bar. Drinking a glass of water before that second coffee of the day. Self-care can be slowing down, refusing to rush, saying no or actively resisting. Healthcare is self-care too, but mums are missing dentist appointments and putting off going to the GP because they can't afford it, or fit it in the schedule, or they're just too tired to organise one more thing. More than 40 per cent of the Angry Mums Club felt poor diet and nutrition contributed to their mum rage. And we know most of us aren't getting enough sleep.

Self-care can also be expensive. Many of us can't justify shelling out for a $70 massage very often (if at all). Same goes for the out-of-pocket costs of regular sessions with a psychologist or physiotherapist, or medications that could help manage our pain or mental health. We're giving up gym memberships to cut costs, thinking twice about feel-good purchases like new clothes or haircuts, or feeling guilty about paying someone to look after our children while we look after ourselves. Angry Mums Club members talked a lot about a lack of 'me time' and 'desperation for a break from children'. A third named the loss of their social life as a factor contributing to their anger in motherhood. One specifically mentioned that she was set off when her co-parent 'prioritises their social time outside the home at the cost of me being the "on" parent at more difficult times'. (Or, you could say, the default parent. More on that later.)

In America, the 2024 State of Motherhood report found 39 per cent of mums got at least an hour to themselves each day.[4] When the National Parenting Pulse Survey asked 8300 Australian mums, dads and carers how much time they got for self-care in 2024, most said they had an hour a day, or less.[5] The survey was run by the Triple P – Positive Parenting Program, which was founded by Queensland Professor Matt Sanders. He told me 56 per cent of mums and 30 per cent of dads were unhappy with the amount of self-care time they got. Learning to take care of yourself while parenting is 'one of the most basic principles' of Sanders' program, which has been taken by more than 375,000 Australians since 2022 – and part of that is knowing that we have a responsibility to 'do self-care non-selfishly'. So maybe don't go to the gym right when your partner is dealing with witching hour, but definitely find what works for you, so you can 'do the kind of parenting you'd like to do'. As he says, 'there's no gold medals for martyrdom in parenthood.' Although, if there were, one of the couples Professor Sanders has worked with would be in the running. He told me they had gone more than four years without a single date night. Somebody send help!

Getting alone time is essential for self-care – and for managing mum rage. But for parents, this can feel as elusive as nabbing the last remaining Elsa dress on the rack, in your daughter's size no less, the day before Christmas. There was a point when my second child reached about nine months old that I realised I couldn't remember the last time I had been alone. We had help with our eldest, halving my workload, but the little fella was almost always within arm's reach – including in the shower, on the loo and while I slept – and I hadn't registered how the constant company was affecting me.

In this context, there is a lot of talk about micro-moments of self-care. You know the type: take five minutes to drink your coffee while it's hot, take a shower alone, feel the sun on your face or the grass underfoot. If you can't do 20 minutes of meditation, try two. Go to bed 15 minutes earlier. Most of these things are low, or no, cost and certainly won't hurt. Sociologist Dr Sophie Brock, who has raised her young daughter as a single mum, encourages us to think about how we can meet our needs while parenting. 'We need to be careful about equating self-care or time to tend to ourselves as being dependent on having space away from our children,' she told me. 'It can look like having a glass of water before you feed your child, or having a plate of food for you, not just picking bits and pieces of leftovers as you're cleaning up. And there have absolutely been moments where a shower has been self-care for me, and going to get groceries alone,' she added with a wry smile. But Dr Brock is insistent that getting time alone for self-care should be an equal opportunity pursuit. Speaking on the *Beyond the Bump* podcast in 2022, she put on notice the dads 'buying their leisure time through mothers' mental loads. It's not okay that dads, or the other parent in the household ... is able to have leisure time ... and mums don't get that.'[6]

I know that many mums don't have an easy support network that enables them to get regular time away from their children. We'll discuss the importance of the village in more detail soon, but for now just remember that yours can look any way you like. If you are short on family or friends who can help, but you have the disposable income, then paid child carers can be part of your village. Can you book a casual day at your childcare centre to get a break? Are there trustworthy teens around looking for extra pocket money? (Even if they just come around to watch the kids while you lie down for a bit ...) Do you live near a gym with an inhouse crèche? Could you arrange with any parents of your child's friends to each host a sleepover? Are your kids old enough to be left at home while you take a 15-minute walk around the block? Or could you make friends with the neighbours and ask them to keep an ear out while you walk? And if you can't be completely alone, is there any sort of mums' group, morning tea drop-in, church session or playgroup where – for the cost of a gold coin – you could take your children and sit back while volunteers keep an eye on them and you finish a cuppa in peace? (This last one was a lifesaver for me.)

It might sound like a lot of hard work but I have come to believe that it is crucial to make the effort, to find any way you can to get *some* alone time (or at least some 'not 100 per cent on' time). This respite is the key to sustainable long-term mental health in parenting, as far as I'm concerned. Learning to ask for help to get some alone time has taken practice and is still a work in progress for me. Dr Brock reminded me that the awkwardness or reluctance we can feel is part of the social construction of motherhood. 'Because asking for help, on some level, can be equated with saying, "I can't do this on my own," and we're supposed to be able to do it on our own, according to the perfect mother myth,' she said. 'So it can be interpreted by some mothers as almost an admission of failure.' It can also be painted as selfish: 'These are your children, it's your responsibility, so it's "selfish" for you to be asking others for help. So often, we don't have that [support] as mothers, so we just keep going and going and going to a place where you feel unrecognisable,' Dr Brock said. 'But you're not selfish for being self-focused. That's actually a gift for you and your children.'

If we can manage to put aside our hesitation in asking for help, and assuming that help is forthcoming, there can still be a challenge in *how* we use it. 'Sometimes it might feel easier to have somebody else take on the care of our children if we're using that time to be outwardly "productive", but what if we were to use that time to have a bath and a nap?' Dr Brock asked. 'Often, a whole new level of guilt arises. This is because the perfect mother myth tells us it's selfish to do things for ourselves.'

This was definitely a problem for me. I first got comfortable with asking the grandparents to take the kids so I could clean at home uninterrupted, or if I had to work late or go to a doctor's appointment. But it was much harder to ask for babysitting so I could go to the gym or just stay home and rest. Only recently have I managed to automate what I call 'Self-Care Saturdays'. It started with an awkward request to my partner: Could I go to the gym on Saturday morning and stay out for a coffee on my own afterwards, while he stayed home with the kids? For the first four or so weeks I received a phone call at some point while I was out. It wasn't a demand to come home, just a question, but it was an interruption and it irritated me. I persisted. I actively resisted. And then one Saturday I was out for two hours and returned home without a phone call. Today, it is an automatic thing – I go out for a bit on Saturday mornings. Or, if I want, I sleep in. But it's my time and my partner has the kids. And I return the favour on Sunday mornings.

Self-care has to be a team effort to be sustainable. There's no point carving out time for you to have a nap or read a book, only for every member of the family to traipse in at some point asking where their socks are or what time dinner will be. Two similar scenarios in our house come to mind here – with two different outcomes. The first happened much earlier on in my mothering journey, the second more recently

The self-care squeeze

after I'd been doing a lot more asking, resisting and axing my guilt. In scenario one, I attempted to have a bath after I thought both our kids were asleep. No sooner had I lowered myself into the steaming water than a child appeared in the doorway. She didn't want to go to sleep alone. Her dad was still awake, so I sent her in to see him. Like a ping-pong ball, she bounced straight back. 'I don't want Daddy.' I returned serve, twice more, but lost the match. I was beyond frustrated and sick of yelling out to my partner in vain. But I was also stubbornly determined to have this bath. So I told my daughter if she didn't want Daddy to put her back to bed she'd have to sit down in the bathroom and wait for me to be finished. Then I stared fixedly at the book I was trying to read, distractedly re-reading the same sentence for about ten minutes while she wriggled around on the bathmat. Eventually, I registered the soft purr of a child snoring. I finished the chapter I was reading, got out and towelled off. Then I carried the sleeping child back to her bed, still steaming from the interruption as much as the water temperature.

In the second scenario, I again drew a bath after we'd put the kids to bed. (It's a self-care staple for me because it helps with my endometriosis pain and I don't have to leave the house.) This time I got to spend about 15 minutes soaking on my own before our daughter appeared in the doorway needing something. I tried sending her off to her dad, who was still awake. She reappeared almost immediately, reporting that he had told her to go back to bed. I'm not entirely sure if that's what happened, or if she didn't even go into our bedroom because it wasn't Dad she wanted. This kind of scenario has previously sent me flying into a rage. *Surely, he can hear what's going on. Why can't he just get up and sort it out, FFS?* This night, I was frustrated but not rageful. I told her she'd have to wait while I got out and dressed. After all that, she didn't seem ready to go back to bed. Instead, she wanted to go outside and see the stars. *Fine then*, I thought, *why not?* So we went into the backyard and I lay down on the wooden deck while she climbed into the trampoline with her torch. I ended up trying to do some deep breathing while she bounced, torchlight shining off the safety net surrounding her. And then a surprising thing happened. Seeing that I was trying to relax, my sweet girl came to sit next to me and began tracing her fingertip around my face, drawing the shape of a butterfly. This is something my mum used to do for me when I was going to sleep, and I've done it with our kids to help them drift off. What, on another occasion, could have turned into a terrible night of frustration and resentment ended up leading to a beautiful moment.

Looking back, there were a few factors that made the difference. I'd probably had enough sleep the night before. I'd eaten dinner. I'd at least got 15 minutes to myself before she appeared in the bathroom. But I also distinctly remember a feeling of surrender. Like, *fighting this is going to require more energy than I have, so let's just go with it*. Remember, we've got to figure out what is worth actively resisting, and what to let go. It was about 9 pm, well past her bedtime, when we finally came back inside and sat down on the couch. I turned on the television and she snuggled next to me while we watched a cooking show until she fell asleep. The whole evening went against all the rules of 'good parenting', but it was good enough.

Hardest of all for me has been asking others to watch my children so I can pursue something just for me. I haven't gone back to regular yoga classes and I don't organise to have dinner with friends after work, even though I desperately want to. Even when writing this book, which began as something just for me, I don't think I would have been able to justify taking the alone time it has required if I hadn't secured a publishing contract. That (relatively small) economic benefit somehow made it easier for me to argue that there was a 'reason' I needed time alone. (I know, I know!) This came up when I spoke with *Mom Rage* author Minna Dubin. She also attributed part of the shift in the division of labour in her California home to her getting a book contract and a deadline. 'It's much easier to say, "I need you to be in charge [of the kids] because I have to work,"' she agreed. 'I've always been a writer but I didn't prioritise my writing to such an intense degree as I did when I had to write this book in one year.' Both Dubin and Dr Brock urge us to consider how we can make space in our lives for creative pursuits. That could be gardening, dancing, cake decorating, applying make-up, brewing craft beer, building LEGO models or anything else that allows us to express ourselves. 'If we don't have space for that anywhere,' warned Dr Brock, 'anger will be a little red flag going, "Hey, remember *you*? Where do *you* exist in your life?"'

But no one is going to offer up that alone time on a silver platter (or not often, anyway). Most of the time we have to carve it out within our circumstances. It's awkward at first, but we have to get over it and ask. And then not feel guilty about it. Because having some time to ourselves really does raise our threshold for the irritating and difficult moments in mothering. Like, for example, the day I finally organised an afternoon to myself and cashed in my Mother's Day massage voucher. My monkey mind started up the minute my face lodged in the little hole at the top of the massage table. *My nose is itchy. Did I remember to lock the car? Yikes, does she have to pull my undies down that much? I wonder what the long-term health effects of chronically high stress hormone levels are ...* Eventually, I settled in and relaxed. Later that night, my partner and I had a testing time with one of our kids, who was being more recalcitrant than usual. For once, their dad was getting more frustrated than me. I stayed calm much longer than I usually would have. It no doubt had something to do with the fact that I'd had that time to myself earlier. It can't always be a spa visit, but offering a struggling mum even an hour to herself is one of the best gifts you can give her.

Burning out

It wasn't until I started researching this book that I heard the term 'parental burnout'. It seems so obvious in hindsight but I'd not previously put the two words together. I'd heard of job burnout, often associated with fields like law, medicine and teaching. Sufferers end up exhausted and begin to emotionally withdraw from their work until eventually they can't go on. The roles where it seems most common are usually demanding, high-pressure, competitive and high stakes. Sound like another job you know? If there were an honest job ad for motherhood it would read something like this:

> On call 24 hours, unpredictable schedule, relentless deadlines, serious consequences for failure to perform, no sick leave or holiday pay, occasional bonus in the form of beaming smiles or handmade cards. Oh, and it's a competitive market but there's no pay bump for doing it better than anyone else.

Under these conditions, it's no surprise that parental burnout can creep up on some of us until, one day, we wake up and just can't do the job anymore.

You might be wondering why I'm talking about burnout in a book about anger. The two seem contrary, right? Anger is volatile and explosive. Burnout feels more like depression or inaction. But we know from earlier chapters that frustration, irritability and outbursts can be signs of depression – and they can be red flags of parental burnout too. A 2018 study of Belgian mothers found some became increasingly frustrated and irritated before a breakdown. One mother, Veronique, told the interviewers that she shouted all the time. Another, Benedicte, revealed her worst moment came when she was tired, wanted to go to bed and began screaming at her daughter to put her pyjamas on. She ended up punching the wardrobe in her daughter's room.[1]

Research on the specific feeling of parental burnout, as opposed to job burnout, has been building since around 2014. Estimates of the prevalence of parental burnout are between 2 and 12 per cent of parents.[2] The Parental Burnout Inventory (PBI) was developed in 2017 by three Belgian researchers to measure three elements in affected parents: exhaustion, emotional distancing from children, and feeling a sense of being incompetent, or less effective, as a parent.[3] About a year later two of these researchers and another colleague developed the Parental Burnout Assessment (PBA). It had four dimensions: exhaustion, emotional distancing from children, feeling fed up with being a parent, and feeling differently about yourself as a parent compared with how you used to. The researchers explained the difference: just because parents lose fulfilment in their role, not all of them stop being competent parents (as was suggested by the PBI definition). The emphasis on contrasting their current parenting with their former parenting (before feeling burned out) was also made to distinguish between 'exhausted parents rather than permanently dismissive ones'. The former can improve their situation with support, the latter may be purposefully neglectful.[4]

There are some key differences between parental burnout and depression or postnatal depression. For example, parental burnout is more often considered when children are older than 18 months, to remove variables more specific to postpartum depression.[5] The depressive mood of parental burnout is also not necessarily felt in every aspect of life, but is specific to the parenting role and tasks.

While researching the topic, I came across the Parental Burnout Facebook group, run by New South Wales–based psychologist and family coach Hélène Gatland. I posted a message about my book and asked burned-out mums to get in touch. Not long afterwards, I got an email from Lucia, a 49-year-old mum of two from Adelaide. A few years back, Lucia woke up three days after Christmas and, as she watched her husband leave for work, called out: 'You can't go in today. You can't leave me with these kids. I just can't anymore!'

A series of compounding issues had led to that moment. Lucia's father had passed away and she had been unable to get to the funeral. Around the same time her family had moved to the city from country South Australia, and the physical restrictions of city life had affected the mental state of everyone in the family. Soon it was the summer school holidays, a long stretch of weeks when, as Lucia described it, 'we were in a new house, limited friends, hours to kill every day'. Her daughter, aged nine, who has an ADHD diagnosis, and her son, eight, were 'doing their usual bickering, moaning, demanding ... One wanted to go out to the park, the other complained it was too hot, you know how it is,' Lucia explained. All this came in the lead-up to Christmas and her stress was building. 'I can remember taking the kids out in the evening and them being very high needs, it all felt so hard. When I came home, I cried as I wrapped the Christmas gifts. My husband heard me and came in to see what was wrong. I said, "It's just not supposed to be like this." There seemed to be so much disharmony. Kids being upset, me getting upset at them through frustration, my husband getting upset at them. It was just a really hard, horrible time.'

In a bid to short-circuit the downward spiral, Lucia booked herself in for an emergency appointment with a GP on Christmas Day to get some anti-anxiety medication. The so-called festive season 'was horrible', she recalled. 'I had nothing in me to give. I felt so awful for my children. I hope they never remember it.' Things continued to worsen in the following days and Lucia stopped eating. The burnout was setting in. 'I was absolutely numb so the kids' bickering didn't even penetrate. My anxiety levels were so high I would pace up and down. I could only sleep about three hours per night.' After Lucia told her husband she couldn't be left alone, he took carer's leave to stay with the kids and Lucia went back to the doctor. She was on annual leave from her job as a teacher but knew she would soon have to return to the classroom. When school went back she lasted a couple of days at work and ended up off again for another two weeks. 'I was so burned out and anxious, I just couldn't do it,' she said.

In total it took a couple of months, and trialling two medications, for Lucia to feel that the tide was beginning to turn. It took a lot longer to understand why she sank so low. 'There were a few factors involved … I wasn't really aware of the impact of each one individually, but I am sure that they didn't make things any easier. I still carry the guilt of that time, my kids seeing me so low, my husband so worried. He had never seen me like that.' By the time Lucia got in touch with me she said she still got overwhelmed and annoyed, but less regularly, and the medication 'stops the spiralling'.

So how do you know if you might be burned out? Well, there's a quiz for that. Created by Professor Moïra Mikolajczak and Professor Isabelle Roskam, who developed the PBA and PBI, it includes 23 statements about parenting and asks users to rate how often they feel that way. The statements include 'I'm so tired out by my role as a parent that sleeping doesn't seem like enough' and 'When I get up in the morning and have to face another day with my child(ren) I feel exhausted before I've even started'. Other phrases touch on being 'completely run down', 'on autopilot' and 'in survival mode'. There are also statements that are hard to read, especially if something inside you were to identify with them, such as 'I can't stand my role as a father/mother anymore' and 'I'm no longer able to show my child(ren) how much I love them'.[6]

I didn't discover this survey until I began researching this book but, on my first go, I filled it in as if I were back at my lowest point. For quite a few of the statements I answered 'every day', including that doozy about being over it all before you've even got out of bed. (Although I have always told my kids I love them every day.) After I pressed submit, a pop-up delivered my results. 'You are one of the parents who is currently in a situation of parental burn-out,' it told me. 'You are exhausted, exhausted, exhausted, exhausted.' (Yes, there really were four exhausteds.) It went on to describe what my life was like back then, as if the researchers had been watching through our front window: 'Sometimes, the mere thought of a new day to face seems unbearable to you ... Feeling guilty because you got angry or angry more than you should have ...'

Then it gave me a blunt warning: 'At this stage, it is crucial for your mental and physical health and/or the well-being of your children that you take a break. A professional can help you better understand how and why you got there, and provide you with directions to help you get back on track. You need to take urgent care of yourself.' When I experienced this, it had taken me much longer than a five-minute questionnaire to figure out what that pop-up told me – that I needed a real break, and a professional to help.

Back to the quiz. I refreshed the screen to complete a new set of answers, based on how I feel now, after seeing my GP and a psychologist, starting medication, making changes at home and working on this book. (And, to be fair, when my children are older, sleeping more and toilet trained.) The difference in result was stark: 'You are not at risk of burning out at the moment.' And it was right. But the pop-up warned me: 'This does not mean that you have never burned out or that you will never burn-out. It simply means that, at the moment, your protective factors are more numerous than your risk factors.'

The pressure to live up to intensive mothering, which we learned about earlier, has been identified as a contributor to burnout. Remember that 2018 study of Belgian mothers? It found that many who ended up burned out had initially 'overinvested' in the role, feeling they must be in charge of everything, execute perfectly, anticipate every need and not ask for help. The five mothers extensively interviewed were aged 30 to 42 and each had two children ranging in age from two to 14. The interviewers found these women went from being willingly and consciously overinvested in mothering to questioning their competence, feeling they were not living up to the standards that they and society had set, and that they didn't have the resources to keep up. From there it was a 'slippery road' down. As they began to feel like failures, they emotionally distanced from their children. Some lost control and verbally or physically lashed out. This was followed by shame, guilt and isolation, on top of exhaustion. By then they were burned out, feeling trapped and failing in their role as a mum but too tired and ashamed to ask for help.[7]

Burnout can lead some parents to harm their children, or feel the impulse to. In a paper titled 'Parental burnout: what is it, and why does it matter?', researchers found that burnout 'strongly increases ... neglectful and violent behaviour towards one's children'.[8] And other research shows this can happen in 'all kinds of families', regardless of education level, income or addictions among parents.[9] However, it's not inevitable. And it's not a straight line between burnout and child maltreatment. Nuanced investigations have found that exhaustion alone is not enough 'to make an initially wellcaring parent more neglectful or violent'.[10] The more important factor is whether they are emotionally distancing from their children, and how badly.

In the paper 'Are all burned out parents neglectful and violent?', researchers surveyed more than 2700 French-speaking parents (80 per cent of them mothers) who had at least one child living at home. The study tracked how symptoms can progress from feeling ineffective or exhausted to disengaging and burning out. The authors argued that to protect children, 'exhausted parents need to be diagnosed and cared for before exhaustion leads to emotional distancing'.[11]

As Belgian mother Elisabeth slid further into her burnout, she more regularly lost control of her emotions when she was with her daughter. She would scream 'hysterically, with a huge violence', she told the authors of the paper 'Parental burnout: when exhausted mothers open up'. She felt that she had no control over the impulse. One afternoon, her child refused to nap so Elisabeth 'dragged her' in bed, knocking her daughter's head. She recalled, 'I suddenly felt an urge inside me to box her to death.' Reading that quote stopped me in my tracks. It is shocking in its honesty and specificity. After imagining harming her daughter, Elisabeth was aghast that she had such thoughts towards her child.[12]

It is important not to brush aside the depth of feeling that comes over some mothers in moments like this. When we think of anger, we might first think of a physical action: shouting, hitting, stomping our feet. But it can also come in the form of intrusive thoughts like the ones Elisabeth was having. Visions of lashing out at her child can burst into a mother's mind. She would never do it, she tells herself, but thinking it is scary and shameful enough.

Research has shown that almost all new mothers experience unwanted intrusive thoughts about accidentally harming their child.[13] Walking down the stairs, they imagine dropping the baby, its tiny form tumbling to the bottom. Pushing a pram down the street, they imagine tripping and propelling the baby into oncoming traffic. Preparing dinner, their mind sees the sharp knife slip from their hand into their infant's soft flesh. Intrusive thoughts about harming children *on purpose* are more common than you might think too. One study found 49.5 per cent of mothers with babies one month old had them.[14] Another found a rate of 44 per cent among mothers of infants.[15] That's right, about half of all new mothers have thoughts like Elisabeth's. They imagine screaming at or shaking their wailing baby, hurling their little body onto the bed or putting a pillow over their tiny face.

But it is not just new mothers who have these thoughts, as the Speak the Secret campaign revealed. It was created by social worker, advocate and author Karen Kleiman, who co-wrote *Dropping the Baby and Other Scary Thoughts*, and founded the Postpartum Stress Center in the US in 1988. On the Speak the Secret website, when I visited in 2024, there were posts from mothers about wanting to run away from home, leaving older children with deserted husbands. One parent wrote: 'Every time I walk past the stairs, my brain tells me to throw myself and/or my daughter down the stairs.' Another described how she walked past her toddler's room and 'thought "I could put a pillow over her face to stop the crying forever". That thought haunts me.'[16]

To be clear, parents don't intentionally conjure up these thoughts or images – the whole point is that they are unwanted and intrusive. They are brief, followed by a hot flush of shame, or horror. Maybe a furious shake of the head to erase the distressing image. And research has confirmed that mums who have these thoughts are *no more likely* to be aggressive towards their child than mums who don't.[17] But have you ever heard such a confession from a mum you know? If you've had these thoughts, have you ever dared to tell someone? Among the Angry Mums Club members 18 per cent revealed they'd had an intrusive thought about harming their child. If we cannot confront this reality, and learn to voice it safely, then we won't ever get rid of the stigma that prevents too many struggling mums from speaking up. Currently, there is just too much risk that an admission of such taboo thoughts – even without any action – would provoke a punitive response.

Crossing lines

After some heavy reading in the last chapter, we might need to take a deep breath here. It's a good time to reiterate that this book is not about condoning mistreatment of our kids. We have a responsibility to keep them safe and treat them with respect, even if we're struggling. However, without the right support and knowledge, anger in motherhood *can* lead to harm to children. No one wants this. No one intends this. But it does happen.

The most common way is smacking. The 2018 survey by the Royal Children's Hospital Melbourne found 13 per cent of parents physically disciplined their kids 'sometimes' and 4 per cent did so 'quite a lot or most of the time'. Unsurprisingly, it was more common among parents with toddlers and preschoolers than older children. There were similar proportions of parents who threatened to use physical discipline even though they didn't follow through (17 per cent sometimes and 6 per cent most of the time). Dr Anthea Rhodes, who authored the survey report, wrote that the findings 'suggest that a significant proportion of Australian parents hold attitudes and beliefs in support of physical discipline'. Half of the 2000 survey respondents believed it was 'unrealistic to think that parents should never use physical discipline'. A quarter felt children 'become unmanageable without physical discipline'. These views often stemmed from parents' own upbringing, with almost 90 per cent saying they had been physically disciplined as children. Despite many believing children needed physical discipline to manage their behaviour, half of parents who used the tactic then conceded, ironically, that they 'often find it difficult to manage their child's behaviour'.[1]

Professor Matt Sanders calls this the 'escalation trap'. (He's the Queensland professor of clinical psychology who developed the Triple P – Positive Parenting Program.) Without the right parenting tools, we can get stuck in a cycle that 'very easily turns into yelling, plus threatening, plus hitting', he told me over the phone. 'What happens is parents ask once, ask twice, their voice raises, it escalates and sometimes, when we're at our worst, children will then cooperate.' (Sounds familiar.) 'Children will also say "Mummy, Mummy, Mummy" escalating and, right at the point when they're at their worst, parents will say "What?!"' (Also familiar ...) The way to exit the escalation trap, Professor Sanders said, is to focus on speaking in a firm, calm voice. 'If necessary, walk away,' he said, 'then go back into the situation and completely start again. It's almost like it doesn't matter what you throw at me, I'm not going to get upset. Basically, no shouting.'

Full disclosure: at this point in the interview, I had to stifle a snort. I just could not imagine being able to parent without ever shouting again. It was also one of those pieces of advice that sounded too simple and obvious to be of any real use. But then I reminded myself that as I've come further along in motherhood, and got a few other mum rage triggers under control, there *are* more circumstances where I've gone to open my mouth to yell and have been able to stop myself. I've taken a deep breath and it has *actually* helped. I've been able to tune out the crying or whinging or fighting or questioning for a second and reset before I did something I'd regret. This is the ideal. But I still can't do it every time. And I definitely couldn't do it at the start of my mission to manage mum rage, when I was too agitated for parenting lessons.

Most of us know when we're crossing a line. If you've picked up this book, it's likely you've said or done something as a mum that you thought you'd never do and you're trying to figure out why, and how to nip it in the bud. I don't support smacking, and certainly not in a premeditated way. I don't want to do it with my children. But I would be lying to you if I said there hasn't been a handful of occasions where, without thinking, I have whacked a little hand reaching for something it shouldn't. This is about my own inability to control my frustration, or to think before I act, rather than an intention to hurt or punish my child. (My thinking brain hasn't been able to get the jump on my amygdalae.) But intentional physical punishment is still happening in Australian households.

The 2023 Australian Child Maltreatment Study found 60 per cent of the 3500 teens and young adults (aged 16 to 24) surveyed could count at least four times they were smacked, hit or otherwise physically punished during their childhood.[2] It has also been shown that it takes only four instances of corporal punishment to increase the risk of developing anxiety or depression in later life. I spoke with Professor Sophie Havighurst, who was the lead researcher on the 2023 'Corporal punishment of children in Australia' report, for my day job at the newspaper.[3] The University of Melbourne researcher told me smacking may change a child's behaviour in the immediate term, but over time they can end up becoming more aggressive. This can lead parents to escalate their discipline to maintain control. Professor Havighurst agreed that smacking can often come from 'an automatic reaction' but argued it should still be made illegal. 'We all have those moments, it's hard being a parent,' she told me for *The Advertiser* article. 'I think mostly people don't feel great about smacking their child. [But] people won't change their behaviour until we change the law.'

South Australian social worker Sally Rhodes told me that justifications for smacking are brought up frequently by parents she works with. 'They'll say, "I was smacked, it never hurt me,"' she said. 'But the issue is around when smacking stops working, what happens next?' Given the strain on the child protection system, she said it is highly unlikely that a child would be removed from their parents 'for yelling on its own', unless it strayed into targeted emotional abuse, name-calling, belittling or obscenities. But authorities do intervene when there is a pattern, such as a child who says they don't want to go home because mum yells too much, or when physical discipline becomes a regular feature.

I also asked Rhodes about those moments when parents have an automatic reaction. She estimated she had seen between 50 and 60 cases over the past two decades where a child had suffered 'unexplained injuries', including cases which might be described as a 'shaken baby'. 'It is a split-second thing that can change people's lives forever,' she said. 'It might be throwing the baby on the bed. Or changing a nappy and the baby is constantly moving and the parent ... just [exerts] pressure beyond what a baby can manage. I don't think it's intentional most of the time and there's massive regret.'

Interviews with parents in the United Kingdom found 'loss of control' and 'rough handling' of babies was 'significantly more frequent' among those who reported feelings of anger in new parenthood. The authors of the 2012 paper 'Postnatal mental health and parenting: the importance of parental anger' interviewed 85 first-time parents. Among them ten women and 13 men reported strong levels of anger towards their baby. These feelings were more common among parents whose babies had trouble feeding or sleeping or cried excessively. More of the angry parents felt an impulse to harm their baby when they cried or woke in the night. They spoke of swearing at their infants and 'having violent thoughts, even though it is just a flash'. One mother said the worst thing she had felt was wanting to throw her baby 'at a wall, out the window'. Another described her feelings as 'quite murderous', followed by 'humungous' guilt.[4]

Again, admissions like these are shocking, uncomfortable, almost unbelievable to read. These things are not meant to be thought about children we longed for and love. But, by now, we know these feelings are not uncommon. Government-funded parenting courses and public awareness campaigns about the harms of smacking are important. We need those tools to help us be the best possible parents. But we also need honesty. About how hard parenting *can* be. About what we might feel when it gets tough. And a safe enough space to be honest if we feel like we're rapidly approaching a line, so we can get help before we find ourselves stuck on the other side.

Ghosts in the nursery

There is nothing like becoming a parent to make you reflect on the way you were parented. Who among us hasn't opened their mouth one day to say something to one of our kids and heard the voice of our own mother or father come out? Or done something from our parents' playbook that we swore we'd never repeat when we had kids? This is not going to be a chapter about how terrible my parents were (they weren't) or how we can blame all our mum rage on those who came before (we can't). But our childhoods are worth examining because they can provide crucial insights.

The first thing to understand is that your motherhood is haunted – or, as child psychoanalyst Selma Fraiberg wrote in 1975: 'In every nursery there are ghosts.' We might not be able to see them but our mothers and fathers, and theirs before them, are all hovering, ready with their habits, advice and judgements. Professor Fraiberg, who was director of the Child Development Project at the University of Michigan, described the ghosts as 'visitors from the unremembered past' of new parents, to whom 'no one has issued an invitation'. Through her work with struggling mothers, Professor Fraiberg observed that the ghosts were most powerful when they were ignored or suppressed. But when mothers acknowledged, remembered and re-experienced the issues bubbling up from their childhood, there was a greater chance that 'the ghosts depart'.[1]

My mum agreed to let me interview her for this book. She said I was a happy baby who would go to anyone, and a fairly 'compliant' child. At one stage, I even sat obediently for a time-out in a room with an open door! Mum doesn't remember me having the kind of big emotions we see in our household now, and certainly not at the same volume (I gave them more grief as a young adult). Although, when she later dug out the handwritten diaries she kept in my early years, she admitted she may have 'forgotten' a few agitations. In return, I don't remember Mum or Dad yelling at me as a kid. It was more of an 'I'm not mad, just disappointed' kind of household. And because I was an only child it was perhaps easier to walk away from conflict and take some space.

But I do have memories of when Mum must have, in hindsight, been grappling with the frustrations of motherhood. I, too, refused to take medicine. Then there was my total inability to empty the dishwasher or walk the dog when asked. My bedroom littered with discarded clothes and wet towels. My entering her study just as she began a work call. Or my best friend and me jokingly referring to Mum as 'Dragon Lady' whenever she got stroppy about something we had (or, more often, hadn't) done. Today, these are in-jokes we can laugh about, but I get how irritating all this would have been. I now understand why Mum would sometimes just go out for the afternoon ...

At the end of the day, though, I had a mothering role model set by a woman who I always knew desperately wanted me, loved me, supported me and would be there for me even if I really messed up. (Same for my Dad, who I know had moments of frustration with his beloved offspring too but would drop anything to help me – and still does.) Later on, it was Mum who warned me about the baby blues, and who came to the hospital when it all fell apart. Today, it's Mum who most often listens to me complain about how bloody hard this gig is. It's Mum who workshopped early plans for this book and (along with others, including Dad) upped her babysitting hours voluntarily so I could get it written. I could rely on my mum when I became a mum, and that's more than what a lot of women I know had.

Some I've spoken to for this book had complicated relationships with their parents. More than a quarter of the Angry Mums Club identified their upbringing as a factor contributing to their anger in motherhood. Quite a few noted they could see how their childhood shaped the mum they became. Eleni, the 34-year-old mother of two from Auckland we met in Part One, has no doubt that the way she was raised has contributed to her difficulties. 'I was a very anxious child and I wasn't parented very consistently,' she said, adding that her parents divorced when she was four. They both remarried and Eleni says she experienced emotional and physical abuse throughout her childhood. 'I remember suffering terribly with anxiety, to the point of getting physical symptoms, and having no way to regulate them and no support or guidance. I would hold it in for as long as I could and then have terrible outbursts, which were just a result of panic and a lack of control. Any time I am overwhelmed [as an adult], I can see the same pattern repeating, but by then I'm so far gone I feel helpless to pull it back.' Eleni told me she'd like to see a counsellor so she 'could blurt out all my thoughts and they wouldn't judge me ... I hope.'

Even if a mum has the clarity to see that unresolved issues from her childhood may be contributing to her anger, it's a whole other thing to find the time and money to see someone about it. The wait for a GP might be too long so they give up. Or they get an appointment but have to cancel because they catch a cold from one of the kids. If they can get to the GP, they can be put on what is known as a Mental Health Treatment Plan, which entitles Australians to up to ten subsidised individual psychology visits and ten subsidised group sessions per year. This entitlement was increased to 20 appointments in response to the COVID-19 pandemic but was cut back to ten at the start of 2023 – a move criticised, understandably, by health advocates. A separate allocation of three counselling sessions is available to Australian women who are pregnant or in the 12 months following a pregnancy. A GP may give a referral but then a mum starts over on a wait list for a counsellor or psychologist with a slot open. They might get the appointment but can't pay the gap fee, or their child care on the day falls through. The choice to opt for a telehealth appointment, through a phone or video call, has dramatically improved options but this is not always available.

And the quality of the help can vary in a system where people usually have to take the first (or only) appointment they can get. For years, Adelaide mum Anna didn't understand how her trauma was affecting her parenting. Her birth mother died when she was a baby and she experienced a series of traumatic events in her childhood, but it wasn't until her eldest child was about 13 that she received a diagnosis of complex post-traumatic stress disorder. 'It makes a huge difference because all of these behaviours that I'm interpreting as my fault and I'm a horrible person, a horrible parent ... I'm not,' she said. 'That is a result of trauma. It's not that the behaviour is okay, but I'm snapping because I'm managing the effects of so much trauma I've got nothing left.' When I visited Anna at home, while the kids were out, she told me she remembers being emotionally explosive as a child but says 'nobody connected the dots' until she found her current psychologist. Now 39, the mother of five experienced postnatal depression following the birth of her first child but, again, didn't receive a diagnosis until years later. She wasn't physically violent but she was 'loud and scary'. There was a heaviness in her voice when she told me she knows she has 'done damage' to her now teenager, who she largely raised on her own in circumstances that would test anyone.

When I asked Anna about her triggers, she said that kids being disrespectful, rude or not listening are top of the list. She recalled times with her eldest when she would 'rant' at him in the car on the way to school. One time at home, she kicked a hole in the wall. 'I was furious so I kicked the wall ... I thought it was solid, but I put my foot through the thing,' she said, rolling her eyes. Anna has also faced challenges raising children who are neurodivergent and gender diverse. Not just the mental and physical health challenges, but the systemic and societal roadblocks they face. There's a lot of fighting for basic needs to be met, and it can be tiring.

When the blow-ups are really bad, Anna often doesn't remember them. She has come to understand this is a trauma response. 'My brain at some point switches off and goes "I'm not remembering this". But then I have this thing where I'm not quite sure if something has happened or not. For the ones I do remember, I will often shut everything down ... and I'll come back to it later and apologise, and try to explain or remake my point in a calmer and actually coherent way.'

A few years ago Anna married into a blended family and says things are less volatile now that she's not solo parenting. She still has outbursts, but she is better at recognising when they're coming. 'I just tend to leave the room because I know I'm overstretched and I can feel the stress and anxiety rising, and I know it's not smart for me to stay,' she explained. 'I get irritated, but I don't get anywhere near the same level.' She and her spouse also have a good sense for when one or the other needs to 'tag out' and which of them is best placed to manage a particular issue with a particular child. I asked Anna if, given all she was dealing with, she could have operated this way when she first became a mum. 'Not with the knowledge I had at the time,' she replied. 'If I'd had a therapist that had been able to diagnose and treat me, then maybe I could have. With the support I have now, there is a lot more hope for all of us.'

Some mums have become so used to a certain way of operating during their childhood that they aren't able to recognise it isn't healthy when they repeat it in parenthood. Clinical psychologist Dr Nicole Williams told me that for some clients 'the work is actually to help them understand that this [level of anger] is a problem'. Many mums have had 'quite scary experiences of anger themselves as children' and when they become parents they are 'so consumed by their own experience of threat that they can't think outside of that', Dr Williams explained. It might be hard to imagine, but these mums can perceive their own children as a threat, a trigger to a nervous system that is already on high alert. If, on top of that, they don't have stable housing, are in a violent relationship or are struggling to put food on the table, then they can feel that talking about their feelings is not high on their priority list.

Social worker Sally Rhodes, who began her career in child protection in 1985, meets many parents who cannot see that the way they parent isn't safe. 'Often people will say to us, "Smacking them with a ruler, that's not violence ... what I had in my childhood was violence." They'll say, "The kids know I love 'em. They know I don't mean it ..." But you can see the kid cowering in the corner.' In too many cases this is history repeating, Rhodes told me. 'It's their world belief because that's how they were parented. All they know is mistrustful, hostile kinds of relationships, so they don't know how to behave in other ways unless they get that support. A lot of people don't know that until they know it. Having a child can completely bring up things that you weren't even aware were there.'

Research has confirmed that trauma can reshape our brains. In fact, you can spot mothers who experienced past trauma from a brain scan. At the University of Massachusetts Medical School, Assistant Professor Sohye Kim and colleagues put 42 first-time mothers into a fMRI machine and showed them images of their own baby, and a stranger's baby, making happy and sad faces. All the mums were from middle- to high-income families, but some had been identified as having experienced unresolved trauma, related to poor attachment with their parents or insecurity as children. The scans showed these mums had a 'blunted' response to their baby's sadness. Their amygdalae (their threat detectors) didn't light up as much as those of mums without a history of trauma.[2]

These mothers had experienced trauma stemming from absence or neglect, but trauma can of course come from physical violence or the threat of it. The grim reality is one in five Australian women or girls have been sexually abused since turning 15. A quarter have been physically abused by a partner or ex-partner. The same proportion have been emotionally abused by a partner they lived with since turning 15.[3] And Aboriginal and Torres Strait Islander women are 27 times more likely to be hospitalised after an assault than other Australian women.[4]

Pregnancy is a time of increased risk as it can be seen by abusers as a threat to their control over a victim. The Maternal Health Study, by the Murdoch Children's Research Institute, looked at 1500 first-time mothers and their firstborn children from early pregnancy to when the child turned four. It found almost one in five women were afraid of their partner before falling pregnant. The same proportion were abused by their partner in the year after giving birth, and one in five also experienced abuse from a partner in the year that child turned four.[5]

When asked to reflect on their childhoods, one in six women and one in nine men say they witnessed violence involving at least one parent.[6] The Australian Child Maltreatment Study found 61 per cent of the population have been neglected, abused (physically, emotionally or sexually) or exposed to domestic violence.[7] Because these experiences are so widespread in childhood, it is no wonder many parents are triggered when they have their own children. Bickering between siblings, disagreements about disciplinary styles, or fighting with a partner can all remind them of the danger they associated, from a young age, with raised voices or hands. They may fear they'll react in the same way as their parents and the constant vigilance required not to is exhausting.

Rates of childhood maltreatment are higher among girls and women than boys and men, but ghosts in the nursery don't just hover over mums. Adelaide father of two Arman expends a lot of energy trying not to be an angry dad. He grew up with a domineering, cruel and violent father. In 2010, after inflicting decades of abuse, Arman's father murdered his mother in front of hundreds of people at the Adelaide Convention Centre. He is serving a 26-year sentence and has never met his two grandsons. But he is still present in the back of Arman's mind, fuelling the 'small voice telling me not to be that guy'. Arman took six months' unpaid leave to be the primary carer of their 10-month-old son when his wife Genevieve returned to work, which gave him more of an understanding of the 'sequence of provocations' of parenting than many fathers who spend limited time with their children during the week. The 37-year-old told me that both he and his eldest boy, aged four, have 'big emotions'. When we met at his CBD workplace he recounted a scenario where his son asks for eggs for breakfast, which Arman lovingly prepares – only to be told by his son that he wants something different.

Or a time his son hit him over the head with a toy vacuum cleaner, hard and with no warning. And of course there are the bedtimes where his son is rolling around, wanting to play, climbing out of bed until finally Arman is done. He will be 'patient, patient, patient' with his boy 'and then I lose my shit'. (Sound familiar?) 'Then I go back 33 years and I remember my dad yelling at me and the thought comes into my head, "Am I recreating the same sort of household that I grew up in?"'

The early days of parenting were extra tiring because Arman would 'overanalyse everything'. And he definitely had the guilt spiral many mums know so well. Now, after a blow-up, Arman works hard to put things in perspective. He knows his son is safe and he is just expressing emotions. 'He stomps down to the bedroom where his mum is, they have a hug and then they come out,' he said. 'In my childhood home there was none of that. You got a beating; you got sent to your room for a few hours and maybe after that Mum would come along and say, "You guys can come out now."'

Being a Black mother in Australia

For some families, the ghosts in the nursery have hung around for centuries. Every First Nations parent lives with Australia's painful history of colonisation by Europeans. The fear and distrust of authorities that it bred remains in the veins of Aboriginal mothers, stoked by the continued removal of their children by the state at a much higher rate than other families. It is an ever-present trigger for anxiety and anger – but it can still take them by surprise.

Like when April Lawrie gave birth to her second son. Born at an Adelaide hospital in 2002, he was a healthy weight, breastfeeding well and ready to go home and meet his older brother. But as Lawrie, a proud Mirning and Kokatha woman, was walking, newborn in arms, to meet her husband down the corridor, she heard a nurse call out: 'Just a minute. You can't leave.' Confused, Lawrie looked down at her sleeping boy and her packed bags. 'Why not?' she asked the nurse. 'Well ... because you're Aboriginal,' came the reply. Lawrie looked at her, dumbfounded. Three days earlier, she had been admitted to hospital to give birth and the fact that she was Aboriginal had not been raised. 'Tell me,' she asked the nurse, 'why is it that being Aboriginal means I can't leave the hospital?' 'Well,' the nurse hesitated, 'because you're a risk.'

This interaction played out more than two decades ago but Lawrie told me it remains common. Now the mother of three adult sons, Lawrie was appointed South Australia's first chief advocate for Aboriginal children in 2018. Back when she had that racist experience in the maternity ward, she was an executive director of Aboriginal Health, within the SA Department of Health, 'sitting at the table with the CEO of the Women's and Children's Health Region'. But to that nurse, she was just another Black mum. 'They just took that I'm Aboriginal and I'm a risk, without wanting to understand who I was, or the fact that I've had a successful birth before. No, all that went out the window because they just saw my culture and my race. I said, "You need to worry about those who have medical risks, because culture is not a risk. I'm going."'

When I asked Lawrie (already anticipating the answer) whether that experience made her mad, she told me she was 'fucking angry. I'm thinking, *How dare they*.' Her strong connection to her culture, her education and her knowledge of the health system meant she was able to push back and leave with her boy, but for too many Aboriginal mothers this is not the case. Lawrie released a scathing report in 2024 about the removal of Aboriginal children into South Australia's child protection system, which included harrowing reports of newborns taken from mothers straight after birth, sometimes without prior warning.[1]

There were 44,866 Australian children in state care in 2023–24, and 19,985 (44.5 per cent) of them were Aboriginal or Torres Strait Islander.[2] Yes, almost *half* of all children in state care are Aboriginal. And in many cases, Lawrie says, it's for things that wouldn't prompt a report about a white family. During her inquiry, Lawrie read case notes on one Aboriginal couple whose young child was removed after a red flag was raised about a suspicious bruise. The child was taken out of their community and observed for days in hospital. Over that time, it became apparent the bruise was, in fact, a birthmark. But Lawrie says written reports about the parents to the courts 'still said that this is a bruise on the child because they had this narrative that the child's been neglected and physically harmed'.

Lawrie suspects a report was made about her as recently as 2023 when she took a young relative to hospital to treat an infection. 'All of a sudden, they started talking to [them] as if I didn't exist. They started asking this child, "Who lives at home? Are there any males there? Do you have your own bed?" and I said, "I beg your pardon!"' Lawrie was incandescent and made a complaint, which drew an apology from the doctor. 'He said, "I don't know why I did that" and I said, "I'll tell you why. Because you have a racist assumption – your training has probably dictated that – that every Aboriginal child that comes in with an infection ... that's abuse,"' she recalled. 'I get angry about that. Lots of Aboriginal women get angry about that. We should not have to second-guess, or work out a strategy to defend ourselves. We should be able to access these services. I get angry because of the injustice in the services that should be helping us, not crucifying us.'

The same fury rose when an older white lady in the street yelled at Lawrie to cover up her baby, and when she was told to stop breastfeeding in a restaurant. 'We're always checking, would you have done that to a white woman?' she explained. 'It's actually about the racist assumptions that people have of Aboriginal women ... whether you are capable, whether you're competent, that you don't know how to look after your kids, that you're all victims of domestic violence. Or that you're neglecting your kids, you're all druggies, you don't send your kids to school, you all starve your kids.'

But showing that anger often makes things worse, playing into a persistent and lazy stereotype. 'You're [seen as] an angry Black woman who is violent,' Lawrie said. 'They don't stop and think, "She's angry because of injustice. She's angry because she didn't get the right service. She's angry because she's being told she can't have her children. She's angry because she's been told that being a victim [of domestic violence] means you can't protect your children."' At the root of the anger is the legacy of colonisation, when Australia's first people were decimated, dispossessed and disrespected by European settlers. 'It's about oppression ... about self-determination and having autonomy.'

Not a single Aboriginal mother I have spoken to for this book has said she would willingly admit she wasn't coping. Certainly not to a stranger, or anyone in a relative position of power. It's not worth the risk. With all my white, well-off, educated privilege, I still felt nervous admitting I wasn't coping, let alone that my inability to cope was showing up as anger. Is it any wonder that Aboriginal women, women of colour, those for whom English is not their first language or those who have experienced trauma don't seek help in a system geared more towards surveillance than support?

'If you're an Aboriginal woman, a mother, a child, you try and make yourself invisible, because you are already highly visible to the system,' Lawrie said. 'Aboriginal women going into emergency departments, going to a GP and looking for help, you know you're going to unsafe places. I know Aboriginal women who are proud Aboriginal women but they don't say it because they know they'll get a different response. They know there'll be eyes on them unnecessarily, that people are looking for a reason for an intervention, rather than going "How can we help you?"'

This view is shared by Eastern Arrernte mum of seven Shona Reid, who we heard from in Part Three. As the Guardian for Children and Young People in South Australia, she also advocates for more than 4800 children living in state care. When I asked her how Aboriginal families can seek help safely, and what that looks like, she said quietly, 'They don't. So it looks like helplessness. It sounds defeatist but it's true. There is nowhere to go, there is no one to see [without risk].' This is what fuels the rage for Reid – the 'shameful' expectation that Aboriginal mothers will lose their children to the system – and the fact that it is a win if 'we've kept our kids … History has created that legacy. We just don't trust anyone.'

Despite what I imagined to be a stressful juggle mothering her kids, who range in age from nine to 31, Reid says she is 'quite a relaxed child rearer. My frustration, my anger, usually is not around the kids, it's usually about someone else's injustice.' She told me how one of her children was accused of skipping the same class at school every week, until the family pointed out that he was attending an Aboriginal cultural activity at that time. She has had to weigh up with her children whether they should wear clothing bearing the Aboriginal flag or other cultural symbols, counsel them after bullying by children and adults, and tell them that they can't go to the park on their own because 'you don't know who you'll run into ... So instead of letting them have the freedom and agency to interact with the world like the rest of Australia's children, you've got to watch them,' she said. 'You have to have conversations with them that other people don't have to have with their kids.'

While she understands the frustrations of the mental load, the logistics of getting everyone in her large family where they need to be and delivering in her paid job, Reid said these issues are weighted differently for Aboriginal mothers constantly butting up against systemic racism and discrimination. 'Other people get to be angry about the everyday living stuff,' she said. 'We have to reserve our anger. Every day we've got to make an assessment ... is this worth the battle today? It's the same anger over and over ... that's what gets exhausting. But maybe that's why I'm so relaxed about the kids. The whole world is angry at them – why should I do that too?'

At times while interviewing women like Reid I found myself thinking a version of: *What have I got to complain about*? I don't have to contend with racism, abuse or intergenerational trauma. I'm not mothering in a warzone, as so many are around the world. I can afford enough nappies and I have people I can call when things get tough. Being mindful of all that I have in my favour can help with perspective: *This is not the end of the world, I can regroup*. But it can also compound the 'guilt' part of that anger–guilt trap we learned about from

Dr Sophie Brock in Part One: *Why am I losing the plot when I'm so lucky?* Nevertheless, I am not imagining my stressors. As we'll see in Part Five, most Australian mums face very real (and infuriating) inequalities even if they are living in, and earning a decent wage in, cities named among the world's most liveable and egalitarian. So many of our triggers come from the systems we mother in, the expectations of both strangers and those closest to us – and the expectations we put on ourselves.

Part Five

The Juggle Is Real

Trying to make it work

It was 5.12 pm on a Tuesday evening when the text message came through. I was in the kitchen, a pan on the stove frying minced beef. My then two-year-old was hovering at my feet and his three-year-old sister was building with Duplo on their play mat. I'd been home with them all day. I was hungry. They were hungry. Their dad was still on his way home from work. I glanced at my phone to see who had messaged me, hoping for once it was just a scammer. Instead, it was a contact who had been keeping me posted about developments in a story I was covering. The text told me a report we'd been waiting on had finally been released. Yep, at 5 pm. Even if I'd been sitting at my desk this timing would have been frustrating. I was due back in the newsroom the following morning but it couldn't wait.

I looked around at the stove, the kids and (forlornly) the front door. Then I picked up my phone and began a series of back-and-forth texts with my contact and my newsroom chief of staff. *In between, I stirred the mince and put some rice in the microwave.* After briefing the chief about the breaking news, I opened the email app on my phone to look at the report my contact had sent over. *Stopped to shoo the two-year-old out of the kitchen and get him a cup of water.* Began drafting a news article in the Notes app on my phone. *Stirred the mince again and poured in some frozen peas.* Took a last read over my hastily typed words and pressed 'send' on an email to the chief. *Retrieved crayons and paper for the three-year-old, who'd become bored with the Duplo.* Forwarded extra quotes, texted by my contact, to add to the article. *Turned off the stove, took the rice out of the microwave and dished up bowls to cool for the kids.* Took a call from the chief, who had questions. *Hung up and chased the two-year-old, who had snuck upstairs.* Texted my contact to get the extra details the chief asked for. *Heard the front door open – thank goodness. Frantically explained to my partner what was going on.* Fired off a return email to the chief with the extra lines from my contact. *Served up bowls for the adults.* Opened my email again to proofread the final article my chief had put together based on my incoming missives. *Inhaled dinner while the kids were quietly eating.* Refreshed my email. *Got the kids' pyjamas out.* Refreshed my email and checked my text messages. *Brushed my daughter's teeth and headed upstairs to read her bedtime stories while my partner wrangled our son.* A final text from my contact came through at 6.51 pm. Bedtime was 7 pm. *Kept glancing (shamefully) at my phone while reading* The Gruffalo. *Lights out.* Went back downstairs to clean up while obsessively refreshing *The Advertiser* website until my article was published. Then I brushed my teeth and fell into bed. The juggle is real.

Just over a third of Australian mums with children aged four or younger work part-time. This includes a fast-growing cohort of mothers of young children aged under two working part-time. Just under a third of mums with kids not yet at school work full-time. As children get older, more mums shift to full-time hours, rising to almost half by the time their youngest kid reaches ages ten to 14.[1]

A major driver of these trends has to be the cost of raising tiny humans. A report by the Australian Institute of Family Studies (AIFS) in 2018 looked at how much having children added to the budget of an Australian couple on a low income. On their own, the adults needed $833 a week to cover basics. Adding one child to the mix added $136 to the budget. Having another child bumped it up by a further $204.[2] So a couple with two children needed $340 extra each week, or $1360 a month, to pay for their choice to procreate. In 2021 Suncorp Bank's 'Cost of kids report' estimated the monthly bill per child to be just more than $3000 to cover everything from food, clothing, education and healthcare to housing, transport, insurance and technology.[3] That was 10 per cent more expensive than five years earlier.

That same year, in the middle of the COVID-19 pandemic, AIFS researchers found one in six Australian parents felt very concerned about their current financial situation. One in five had recently needed to ask for financial help from family or friends because of a cash shortage. And 16 per cent had not been able to pay gas, electricity or phone bills on time. 'I struggle every week to put food on the table and meet basic needs,' one 39-year-old mum said. 'By the time childcare, school fees, kids' food and needs are met there is nothing left.' A 43-year-old who was the sole earner in her family said uncertainty around finances put 'a lot of strain on our relationship'.[4]

Financial insecurity and the anxiety it generates chip away at a person's ability to keep a lid on their emotions.

The ABS Personal Safety Survey has found rates of partner violence and emotional or economic abuse are far higher in households with 'cashflow problems'.[5] The Reily Foundation's Nadia Bergineti advocates for South Australian parents who have had their children removed by authorities; more than 80 per cent of them are financially insecure. 'I definitely see where parents have the risk of losing their home, being homeless, and it has impacted how they were feeling and the anger they felt in themselves, to not be able to provide for their family,' Bergineti, who co-founded the organisation, told me. 'They are able to reflect that they were shorter with their kids ... and to see the impact that not having money had on their wellbeing, and how that was displayed towards their kids.'

This was also borne out in the 2024 National Parenting Pulse Survey. At least two in five parents of varying socio-economic backgrounds said the rising cost of living had made it harder to be 'a calm, loving partner or parent'. A third said it had affected their relationship.[6]

The proportion of Australian couples where both parents work outside the home rose from 55 per cent in 1990 to 71 per cent in 2022, as tracked by the AIFS. Conversely, the proportion of households with a stay-at-home mother shrank from just over a third to one in five over the same period. But, as we learned back in Part One, the number of stay-at-home dad households has never passed 4 per cent.[7] Men are still demonstrably reluctant to even *reduce* their paid working hours to accommodate their children, let alone abandon earning altogether. (And it seems their employers are of a similar mind ...) The 'Fathers and work' report, released by the AIFS in 2018, found the proportion of partnered dads choosing to work part-time hardly budged either, rising from 6 per cent in 1991 to 10 per cent in 2016. (Among single fathers, the percentage rose from 8 to 15.)[8] The 2025–26 Australian federal Budget features a stark graph revealing that this pattern persists a decade later. It shows a blue line for fathers' work patterns in the first five years after they became a dad that meanders across the middle of the page. In contrast, red lines representing the situation for new mums plummet under the 'full time days' heading and surge upwards under 'part time days'.[9] This is despite Australian workers having a legal right to ask for flexible work arrangements to care for children, regardless of gender.

Adelaide dad Ben would have liked to drop back his work hours when his sons were born, but without decent paid leave on offer at the time, he and his wife would not have been able to sustain it financially. Years later, though, Ben was forced to make a change after he was seriously injured in a near-fatal car crash caused by another driver.

He sustained a brain injury, which affected his executive functioning – arguably one of the most crucial skills in parenting – through damage to those areas of the brain that we learned in Part One of this book help us to organise, make decisions and override our emotional impulses. 'Basically, your filter,' Ben explained. Prior to his injury, those who knew him would have described Ben – who works in a fast-paced industry – as 'very calm under pressure and measured', he said. These days his ability to think on his feet is 'not as strong as it was' and his threshold for 'losing it is a lot lower … I used to be quite good juggling the unexpected or curve balls but now stuff from out of the blue rattles me far more than it ever did,' he said. A day spent at home with his boys, aged eight and five, is often 'more taxing than just about any day in the office ... The kids are the most unpredictable thing in my life. They throw curve balls left, right and centre. So I'd be kidding myself if I didn't say the element of just spending more time around them has an impact too.'

Ben's experience adds weight to my theory that it is time spent with kids, rather than gender or title, that raises our likelihood of experiencing frustration and anger in parenthood. When he used to work long hours in an office, five days a week, Ben would look forward to coming home and spending time with his sons before bed. Now, after going through an extended and uncertain period in hospital and gruelling rehabilitation, Ben is back working three days a week, including a day from home – and he has to pick his battles at bedtime.

'There are some times after putting them to bed when I have to remind myself they're just kids. I unnecessarily blow up at them far more easily than I ever did previously. When I come down from that, I think, "They did not deserve that." I get this wave of perspective ... and I'm like, "What was that even over?" I feel bad because I like to think that I probably would have handled it differently prior to the injury.'

Like me, Ben has also come to understand that a crucial part of managing the rage rollercoaster is in repairing. 'Initially, I would be so appalled at myself [for blowing up]. Then it got to the point where if I carry on, yell and scream or whatever, and the kids start in with the "I hate you, Dad," I'll wait for things to calm down a little bit and then say,

"Well, mate, I'm sorry about before." I sometimes feel pretty shit about the fact that I'm not pulling as much weight as I would like [with the kids] but the great irony is that overall I'm probably doing more now than what I otherwise would have been.'

Ben may be a bit of an outlier when it comes to cutting back his work hours in fatherhood, but the fact that he was pushed to do so by an outside factor is far more common. Research on Australian and American dads has found that among those staying home with their kids just one in five are there purely by choice. The American dads were more likely to state disability, illness or trouble getting a job as the main reason.[10]

Among Aussie stay-at-home dads, surveyed as part of the Growing Up in Australia study, only a fifth said they were the primary carer by 'preference'. More than half gave other reasons similar to their American peers.[11] Experts note Aussie dads are more likely to use 'modified schedules or remote working arrangements' to fit child care around work, rather than give up paid hours.[12]

On the flip side, some dads, and mums, who go back to paid work don't actually want to, but economic circumstances mean they don't have a choice. Their job may be a major trigger for mum rage – shift work robbing them of sleep or manual labour causing aches and pains – but they need the pay cheque. Often dad is the first to return, for myriad reasons we'll get to shortly, including because he likely earns more. In certain families one parent (more often dad) may earn enough that the other (more often mum) doesn't need to work to cover costs. This is a dream for some, who welcome the opportunity to leave the workforce for what they see as the most important job in the world and a guaranteed front-row seat to their child's every developmental milestone. The stay-at-home parent trades pay scales, key performance indicators and annual reviews for flexibility ... as an unpaid, on-call taxi driver, butler, chef, cleaner, nurse, personal assistant, tutor and accountant. Various analysts have attempted to put a figure on what this combined role would be paid if it attracted a wage. In 2021 Salary.com estimated, based on answers from 19,000 American mums about how they spend their days, that it would be worth more than AUD$286,000 a year.[13] But so many mums tell me they feel like this mammoth contribution is rarely recognised by their partners as being as important or necessary as paid work. They too are enraged when their significant other talks about all that 'time off' they get while they're home with the kids.

But going back to paid work can prompt some equally incendiary remarks. Mums are asked, 'How do you do it?' far more often than the dads working alongside us. Sydney-based journalist, author and mum Annabel Crabb gave us an answer in her 2014 book *The Wife Drought: Why women need wives and men need lives*. Why aren't working dads asked how they do it all? Wives, that's why. Crabb urges us to see 'wife' as a role that one person (still usually a woman) plays in a partnership, doing all the things that enable the other person (still usually a bloke) to go on working, earning and succeeding. Or, you might say, having it all. Crabb discusses other common questions that can trigger rage for working mums, including some version of 'Where are your kids?'; if you answer with 'They're with their father', then the classic follow-up is 'Aren't you lucky?' 'Usually, she does feel lucky,' writes Crabb, while lamenting that luck has to be involved for us to find ourselves in an equal parenting partnership. 'But she might also feel a little stabby.'[14] Quite.

Many of us spent years building careers that defined or reflected our identities, that gave us status and stimulation. I get more than a wage from my job and never considered not going back after kids despite the challenges. Industrial relations and gender expert Professor Marian Baird told me there is a 'well established' pattern among Australian mothers. 'Women work full-time, they have their child and then they go back to work part-time,' she said. 'It has almost, I would argue, become a social norm ... a motherhood expectation in Australia.' Professor Baird, who along with her colleagues literally wrote the book on how Australians manage work and care responsibilities, said more women are achieving higher levels of education, have seen their mothers in the workforce and 'expect to have a long-term career'.

Despite expecting things to go this way, University of Sydney–based Professor Baird's research has shown that women who want to have children are often torn between being a great mother and a great worker. 'They're both full-time jobs,' she said. And she was speaking from experience, having, with her husband, raised four children who are now adults aged 35 to 41. At one point they were managing four kids aged six and under. She remembers being exhausted and having 'lots of big discussions' with her husband about why her career stopped and his was going ahead. She also had an internal struggle because she was going against the model of generations prior. 'It was thinking: "My mother never did this. Should I be doing it?" My mother would say, "Why do you put yourself under so much pressure?" And she would say, "You need more rest," which was probably true.' Despite all this, Professor Baird was determined to continue working part-time because 'if you don't keep your foot in the labour market it's really hard to get back in later … I don't think I did the work terribly well, to be honest,' she reflected, 'but it was enough.' (It is comforting to hear this from a woman who has gone on to such success in her field, including being awarded an Order of Australia for outstanding services to improving the quality of women's working lives.)

The struggle to balance work and family responsibilities was the top concern among more than 480 mums, in 20 countries, who responded to motherhood studies sociologist Sophie Brock's call for insight into the difficulties of returning to work after parental leave. Her 2024 survey Mothers at Work revealed the second most pressing issue was securing, paying for and managing childcare. Guilt came in at number three, followed by sleep deprivation and the logistics of breastfeeding or pumping and storing milk on the job. Dr Brock said the results show mums 'are caught in an unsustainable balancing act between career and family. Working mothers are facing a crisis of unsustainable expectations and inadequate support. They're battling exhaustion, guilt and workplace cultures that often undervalue their contributions. It is time for a dramatic shift.'

Other polls reflect similar trends. The 2024 National Working Families Survey of more than 6200 Australian parents and carers in paid work found three-quarters of women and almost 60 per cent of men felt stressed by the juggle. (This was up from 51 per cent and 34 per cent in 2019, pre-pandemic.) Almost 30 per cent of mums and dads had considered leaving their job in the next year because of the clash.[15] And among my Angry Mums Club, half identified work–family conflict as contributing to their anger in motherhood. Examples could include sitting down to help with homework and receiving a work-related call you can't ignore, having to get out the laptop after everyone else is in bed to finish the work that didn't get done in part-time hours, being asked to work weekends or change a shift at short notice, or seeing mistakes have been made because you weren't there to oversee something. Any of that ring a bell?

Technology and the work-from-home culture spurred by the COVID-19 pandemic have given many parents increased flexibility. (In our home it has certainly led to an increase in incidental housekeeping by my partner when he is on a break.) But it also means work can invade every moment of our life – if we let it. I know that, for me, being torn between incoming work information on my phone and a kid begging for a snack or refusing to go to bed has been a common mum rage trigger. I've enabled access to my work email on my phone but have actively resisted turning on notifications. Given my hours can change at short notice if I'm home with a sick kid, and I don't expect others to keep track of my part-time schedule, I always have my email out-of-office response on, with clear details about when I'm working next and who to contact in the meantime (automation: tick). I could be a lot better at screening calls or leaving work-related texts unopened, but curiosity or anxiety usually gets the better of me. I am far more disciplined now, though, about how much of my brain I devote to work when I'm not there and, more importantly, axing the guilt about not being 'on' all the time.

That's work interfering with family time. But family intervening with work can be just as problematic. Australian Bureau of Statistics data shows that women are more likely to miss out on job opportunities altogether because they are shouldering the majority of the child-care load. Remember that stat about 45 per cent of women who wanted a job being unable to take one because of child-caring responsibilities? That was almost six times the proportion of men who were held back from entering the labour market or increasing their hours because they had to look after their kids. (Although, even the statisticians caution that there is a fair level of uncertainty about the men's figure.)

In America, the 2024 'State of Motherhood report' found that two-thirds of mothers had considered leaving the workforce because of the cost and difficulty of finding appropriate childcare. And a third of those aged under 30 made the decision not to have any more children because of the combination of financial pressure, lack of support and 'the need or desire to work'.[16]

If a mum has re-entered the workforce, she is still far more likely to be the one who stays home when a sick child needs care. An AIFS report back in 1991 found mums of preschool-aged children did so 57 per cent of the time, and fathers only 7 per cent. Other relatives, especially grandparents, were more likely to step in than dads.[17] More recent research by the AIFS in 2018 found not much has changed. While stay-at-home mums played nurse to a sick child 91 per cent of the time, stay-at-home dads, bafflingly, still only assumed the role half the time. In homes where both parents worked, sick days fell to mums in almost two-thirds of cases.[18]

A related scenario that strikes fear (and often rage) into the heart of a working mum is the unexpected phone call, be it from childcare, school or a co-parent. I'll never forget my first Saturday back at work after returning from maternity leave. My partner drove me to work, with our daughter, then about 13 months old, in her capsule on the back seat. I waved goodbye to them at 9 am and went to my desk. At about 9.30 am, my phone rang. It was my partner. 'Can she eat cheese?' he asked. Now remember, *our* daughter was 13 months old. By this point she had eaten cheese on countless occasions. There were photographs of her eating cheese. 'Of course she can eat cheese,' I told him breathlessly. I'd not been at work for more than half an hour and I was already having to parent remotely. The mum rage was starting to flare, so I did my best to get off the phone quickly. My partner argues it was better to be safe than sorry, and I suppose he might be right. In later chapters we'll look more at what prompts this kind of second-guessing by dads, and how it can contribute to the default parent scenario that lumps mum with so much of the mental and physical load. (Hint: gatekeeping mums can be part of the problem.)

If we do go back to paid work, it appears that our hours in the office, on the shopfloor or on the road don't hugely change the amount of time we spend with our kids. AIFS analysis of Australian families with four- and five-year-old children found mums who worked fewer than 16 hours per week 'appeared to spend no less time with their child than mothers who were not employed'. Those who worked more hours spent less time with kids from morning to afternoon, but in the evening 'there was little indication of work hours making a difference'. In contrast, longer work hours for fathers reduced time with kids in the evening.[19]

Whether mums are going back to paid work or not, it can feel like a bit of a raw deal. Either way, we seem to lose out on income, superannuation, sanity or respect. So exactly how much is this no-win scenario really costing us?

The motherhood penalty

You've probably heard of the gender pay gap, but have you heard of the motherhood penalty? Read on and prepare to be enraged. The average gap between all men's and women's earnings in Australia is almost 22 per cent. So for every $1 the average man makes, an average woman earns about 78 cents. Over the course of a year the difference adds up to $28,425.[1] The Workplace Gender Equality Agency in 2025 found three out of every four Australian employers with more than 100 staff had a gender pay gap of more than 5 per cent in favour of men.[2]

These numbers illustrate the disparity between all men and women, including a larger cohort of highly paid male CEOs and a greater workforce of lower-paid employees in female-dominated care industries. This might make you resentful enough. But now we need to talk about what happens when those men and women become parents. When a baby arrives it drives a wider wedge between mum and dad, in the form of a 'mommy tax', according to American Ann Crittenden, a former *New York Times* economics reporter and author of *The Price of Motherhood*. Back in 2001 she laid out the financial evidence that mums were being stiffed through the devaluing of their work at home *and* any work they did for pay.[3]

Analysis by Australian Treasury officials has, rather depressingly, found that 'entering parenthood has a large and persistent effect' on the gender pay gap – slashing mothers' earnings on average by 53 per cent in the first five years.[4]

Another illustration of this motherhood gap comes from Princeton University economist Henrik Kleven and his colleagues, who tracked wages and hours worked for childless workers and parents in Denmark (a country praised internationally for its gender equality).[5]

In their analysis, the earnings of Danish men and women are actually about equal in the year before the arrival of a first child. But then women's wages nosedive (even before the baby is born) and by the time the child is one, a giant chasm has widened between mums' and dads' pay. There is a slight uptick in mums' wages in the second year of the child's life (presumably as mothers return to paid work from maternity leave), but then earnings plateau and never threaten to close the gap with the unencumbered dads. Fathers' wages, incidentally, do not change much at all over the decade after having a child. The pattern is similar when looking at the number of hours mums and dads work, but the drop for women is not quite as steep. So, way less pay, but not way less hours ...

More infuriating, though, is a comparison of two data sets from the Princeton University research. One shows how starkly women's wages diverge depending on whether they have children or not. The other shows how men's wages don't budge regardless. I find myself having to zoom in on my computer screen to discern the minuscule difference on a graph between the wages of fathers and childless men in the decade after one has a child and the other continues unhindered. In contrast, you can't miss the Grand Canyon between the sustained wages of childless women and the freefall in pay for their female colleagues who have kids (presumably due to career breaks, part-time hours, discrimination, etc). This is the motherhood penalty in action. And it gets more depressing the more kids you have. Over the first decade of parenthood, the Danish mums of one are able to claw back closest to a dad's wage. But with every child the gap gets bigger.

The Angry Mums Club members haven't missed this. Not all 200 mums in the Club work for pay, but a quarter of them felt that the career interruption or barriers that came with having children contributed to their anger. Professor Marian Baird told me most women have 'absorbed and accepted' that – at least for a period of time – there will be a career downside to going part-time. Australian women know all about disadvantages like the gender pay gap, lost superannuation savings due to taking unpaid leave and missed opportunities for promotion. 'They're very aware of it,' she said, 'but the resentment [about it] is more of a private conversation. They don't get tapped on the shoulder for that role or they don't get that client, and that can come out as resentment against your boss, your peers, your partner ... the world.'

There are exceptions. I know women who have been promoted while pregnant or *on* maternity leave, and while working part-time (including me). Some recent policy changes are promising, like a federal government commitment to pay superannuation on paid maternity leave from July 2025.[6] There is hope this will help to close the super gap that currently leaves Australian women with an average $57,000 less in retirement savings than men.[7]

But for too many mums or mums-to-be, decisions about how long they can take off paid work, when to return and in what capacity are clouded by anxiety, insecurity or pressure. And this is despite legal protections that have been in place in Australia for decades. According to the Fair Work Ombudsman, an Australian worker cannot be fired or demoted because they are pregnant, taking parental leave or have caring responsibilities. They 'should' be able to return to the same job they had before going on parental leave. If an employer is making significant changes to the workplace that would affect the role or pay of someone on unpaid parental leave, they are 'required to take all reasonable steps' to talk to the staff member first.[8]

However, these protections do not always work against more subtle forms of discrimination. Even before having children, there are plenty of women who believe they have missed out on jobs, opportunities or promotions, simply because they are of child-bearing age. And then there are the mums who come back to find things have moved on without them. One Sydney mother I interviewed confided that she was let go less than a year after returning to her role following the birth of her first child. 'Things were really different,' she said. 'My job was being done by someone else ... I'd been back for eight months and then I was made redundant.' The woman, whose children are now 13 and ten, said about a third of the women in her mothers' group were also made redundant after returning to their pre-maternity leave roles. 'There's no coincidence there. We were all professionals, not in junior roles ... and we'd been sort of edged out. Forced out, really. It seems quite clear that going and having a baby does affect women's careers.'

It is especially enraging when a parenting gap in a mum's CV is seen by employers as a liability or a weakness, when we know that motherhood actually broadens our expertise. One mum in the Angry Mums Club told me she had spent two years applying for roles 'with no success' after taking 11 years out of the job market to raise her kids. 'I haven't lost my knowledge or my skillset,' she exclaimed. When this came up during my chat with sociologist Dr Sophie Brock, she said there is value in 'seeing our transition to mothering as a gaining of skills'. It throws us in the deep end, but this can be 'a catalyst for self-exploration and self-growth'. I am unequivocally a better journalist now, having overcome challenges and been exposed to a set of life experiences that have made me more empathetic, informed and curious. I'm also more efficient because I can't afford to second-guess myself as much. Not at the cost of $1 for every minute I'm late to childcare pick up!

Default parent mode

'They grew inside you.'

'You're breastfeeding.'

'You've got that maternal instinct.'

'Mums are just better at this stuff.'

These are a few of the most common reasons people will give when you ask why mum becomes the default parent. We know by now that in Australia and many other countries mums are far more likely to be the one staying home to raise kids (especially in the beginning). This means we are usually the one to do all the early learning and experimenting required to become expert in how a baby likes to go to sleep, what foods they might be allergic to and what size clothes they're wearing. This pattern develops in non-biological families too. On the surface, it seems to make sense: whether we made our kids out of a combination of cells or we were the one to hold them through their first nights after coming to live with us, there is no shortage of evidence that the attachment between mother and child is emotionally and chemically strong.

Researchers in 2013 conducted an experiment that proved what I have long tried to explain to my partner. Scientists at the National Institutes of Health scanned the brains of nine women and nine men, half of whom were parents, while they listened to white noise periodically interspersed with the sound of a hungry baby crying. The second the women heard the infant, their brains lurched to attention. The men carried on listening 'without interruption'.[1] Is this not exactly what happens in so many homes between bedtime and sunrise? Women become the default because we find it biologically harder to ignore the sound of a child in distress!

A separate study of 14 birth mothers and 14 adoptive or foster mothers by University of Delaware researchers found they all reacted equally strongly to images of their own children (biological or adoptive), compared with their reaction to the images of children of strangers.[2] And a Yale University Child Study Center experiment involving 41 foster mothers with infants in their care found similar patterns of hormone increase and bonding as in birth mother and child pairs.[3]

Still, being the mum does not make us the only, or always the best, option. It is becoming clear that much more of mothering is learned, and earned, and dads can do that too. Writing in the *Sydney Morning Herald* in 2018, dad and author Christopher Scanlon put it simply: 'the test of fatherhood is not how involved you want to be, but by how involved you are when you'd prefer to be doing something else'. He added: 'If you're not fundamentally changed by fatherhood, you're not doing it right.'[4] Indeed.

Mounting research is showing that dads' brains *are* changed by parenthood. A 2023 experiment involving 20 Spanish and 20 American men found significant changes in their brains after the birth of their first child. Their brains were scanned while their partner was pregnant and again after the baby reached six months of age. The brains of 17 childless Spanish men were also scanned. Among the dads, there were changes in regions of the brain related to visual processing, attention and empathy for the baby, which were not seen in the non-dads.[5]

This builds on findings from 2014, when University of Denver developmental neuroscientist Pilyoung Kim gave 16 new fathers MRI scans when their babies were two to four weeks old and again between three and four months of age. Dr Kim found the dads' brains changed in ways previously noted in mums, with growth over time in areas related to attachment, mood regulation and the ability to interpret and react appropriately to a baby's behaviour.[6]

Another 2014 study, out of Israel, showed brain changes in fathers as a result of assuming a primary carer role. The researchers examined 89 first-time parents: 20 biological mothers, 21 biological fathers, and 48 gay fathers who had a baby through a surrogate and became primary carers. They found there was a 'global parental caregiving brain network' that was largely the same across all parents and involved parts of the brain related to vigilance, motivation and reward, social understanding, empathy and our ability to prioritise. While acknowledging that birth mothers undergo 'powerful' biological changes that prime them for parenthood, it was 'actual caregiving behaviour' that contributed to the parental brain, the authors concluded. By taking an active role in parenting, through 'practice, attunement and day-by-day caregiving', anyone may activate that network.[7] There it is again: it is the time you spend with the kids – not your sex, gender or title – that makes you a parent.

Default parent mode

This is why it is crucial for mums not to internalise the message that we have to do it all. The earlier dads or partners get elbow deep in the mundane and messy minutiae of parenting, the better – for everyone. This also means mums need to quit the kind of gatekeeping that can block dads out – or we need to realise we're doing it in the first place (awareness first, remember?). Every father I've spoken to for this book (including my partner) has reflected on how being repeatedly questioned, judged or told they're 'not doing it right' erodes their confidence and leads to that kind of second-guessing behaviour I mentioned earlier, in the 'Can she eat cheese?' phone call. Or to some giving up altogether. But 'good enough' has to be good enough for dads too.

There is one place where I found being the default parent to be an advantage, and that was in the hospital after giving birth. For the first five days of their lives both my children were, by default, baby Novak. Their father and I haven't got around to getting married yet (not that I plan on changing my surname either way), so it wasn't until we completed the official paperwork and headed home that they assumed his last name. Otherwise, being the default parent can be a pretty draining experience. (And a shout-out here to all the single parents who are, by default, the default.) If the baby wakes up in the middle of the night, who's the go-to? The default is usually mum, with her in-built milk machines. Or mum, because dad has to get up early to go to work. When the child is lost at the play café, which parent gets the call on the PA? 'Can Jimmy's mum please come to the front counter?' And if the kid has an accident at school, who's getting the call? The default is usually mum, because she's likely the one who filled in the enrolment forms and her name ended up in that prime spot alongside 'Parent/Caregiver 1'.

We've had some default parent doozies in our house. For a while, our daughter refused to let her father put her to bed. For nights on end, I had to listen to her yell, 'I only want Mummy' at her poor dad for about half an hour. I resisted, and he persisted, and now we usually alternate. On the morning I wrote this chapter, my partner had to carry our son out of our bedroom as he wailed 'Muuuuuummy' while I tried to go back to sleep. I'd been woken first by him at midnight to change wet pyjamas and bedsheets. Then two hours later by his sister who needed medicine, water and also a change of sheets. I'd had enough sleep the previous night, I'd had some alone time the day before and I knew my kids needed help, so I remained calm. I also know now that, after a night like this, I will need to catch up on sleep in the morning (if it's possible) or go to bed early the next night to avoid a mum rage build-up. I have finally axed the guilt about asking my partner to get up when the children wake after interrupted nights so I can go back to bed for an hour or two. This might seem obvious, but it is actually a monumental shift for me.

Among the Angry Mums Club more than a third said being the default, or having a child refuse to go to another parent, was a mum rage trigger. Lani, 49, told me her husband was involved 'but even if he is in the house, the first name my kids call is "Mum"'. Genevieve, the Adelaide mum of two boys in her late 30s, gave me a similarly relatable example: 'I could be in the kitchen with one kid hanging off my leg and the other one asking me to do something and their dad, who is a perfectly hands-on dad, is standing there all on his own. And they're still at me instead.' We know Genevieve's husband Arman spent an extended period of time as the primary carer for their eldest son, but it still did not appear to confer him with default status. 'When I was home with him, I don't remember him acting out the way he did with Gen. He just behaved differently with me,' Arman said.

I've been spending a lot of time trying to figure out how couples like Genevieve and Arman, and my partner and me, end up in this situation. Because on this, we *were* warned. If you were born any time from the 1980s onward it's likely you were raised (as I was) to expect a partnership in parenting. After everything our predecessors fought for, we had the impression we wouldn't still have to wage the war. But the data is clear – we're not there yet. So I have struggled when reading some books on the difficulties of motherhood in which the authors seem to argue the unequal distribution of care work is a problem – just not in their household. Their partner is one of the good ones. Fathers are doing more than they used to. These things are also true in my household. But the lopsided, default nature of parenting persists bewilderingly under our roof too. And actively resisting a backwards slide still feels like a daily negotiation.

American author, poet and mother Adrienne Rich openly grappled with this piece of the puzzle in her 1976 book *Of Woman Born*, writing about her husband: 'Whatever I ask he tries to give me ... but always the initiative has to be mine'.[8] Two decades later Sharon Hays found among the sample of American mums she interviewed the common complaint that even if dads are 'willing to help, frequently they must be told precisely what to do'.[9] And American academic and mum of two Nancy Reddy noted another 30 years later in *The Good Mother Myth* that every time she asked her husband for help 'he did it', but they never had a discussion about how they would divide the labour of parenting before the babies arrived.[10] I relate when she talks about watching her husband go back to bed after waking to go to the toilet, while she was 'a chord of flame' trapped under their feeding newborn. American psychologist, author and mum of two Darcy Lockman also tells it like it is in her book *All the Rage*. She interviewed mothers who expressed 'intense disappointment' in their relationships, 'persistent underlying' anger at the fathers of their children and 'dampened sexual desire'.[11] She perfectly articulated my resentment at being stuck in default mode through her own experience: 'I cannot recall … at what juncture watching my husband start to eat while I once again cut up our toddler's food became enough to leave me aggrieved for hours.'[12] Lockman also grapples with the question that nags at me – how do we do more than just acknowledge the imbalance, take some smug satisfaction in being the martyr, or complain about it? How do we shift it? Lockman, Reddy and I have all come to a similar conclusion: that it requires more awkward conversations, and active resisting, than many of us have been doing until now.

On reflection, the default dilemma grew in our household from a mix of physiology and anxiety. Physiology because I breastfed, and never really asked my partner to do overnight bottle feeds (which, in hindsight, might have been a subconscious attempt to live up to the perfect mother myth). As a result, I felt I had to be physically present most of the time. And anxiety because I'm a worrier and I didn't want to

Default parent mode

let the kids out of my sight. Until I did ... and then I couldn't because I had become the default. I didn't become the primary carer because my partner earned a bigger pay packet but I was entitled to take a year off while my boss held my job, and I was eligible for paid leave from both my employer and the government. (I did also *want* to spend time with my babies.) In contrast, because of the seasonal nature of my partner's industry and working for a small business at the time, he was only able to take a few weeks off when each of our children arrived.

The right to unpaid parental leave of up to a year was granted to Australian mothers in 1979.[13] It was expanded to include adoptive mothers in 1985 and fathers in 1990. Paid parental leave was not approved until 2010 and took another year to roll out. At first, it provided 18 weeks' pay to a child's primary carer at the national minimum wage (which in 2025 was $948 for a 38-hour week before tax).[14] The payment is subject to eligibility criteria including maximum income, minimum work hours and Australian residency. Another two weeks – initially dubbed 'Dad and Partner Pay' – was added in 2012, bringing a family's total allocation to 20 weeks. (The name of that payment in itself should tell us something!)

After extended debate and lobbying, changes to the scheme were made to make it more flexible and encourage greater shared take-up. Since July 2023 parents have been able to share 16 of the 20 weeks between them, rather than it being attached only to the primary carer.[15] Two weeks were quarantined for each parent, but the remainder could be used in increments of as little as one day at a time or in larger blocks, and over a two-year period. The full 20 weeks have also been made available to single parents who previously missed out on the Dad and Partner Pay. Since then the total leave allocation has incrementally increased to 26 weeks by 2026.

At the time of the 2021 Census about one in five eligible mothers were on the scheme – but just *one in 100* eligible fathers were getting Dad and Partner Pay.[16] This is where the default starts for many. Dads and partners taking up that payment had to take two weeks off work without their regular pay. When they did that, they were instead paid by the government at the minimum wage. Sure, mums were too, but we already know the gender wage gap in Australia means men are more often the higher wage earner in a family. Many dads either earn too much to be eligible for the payment, or see the minimum-wage offering as a disincentive to taking time off right when a family needs to outlay expenditure on a new member.

The 2024 National Working Families Survey found nearly half of Australian dads took less than a month of parental leave for their youngest child – whereas more than 90 per cent of women took more than four months. The main reason for the contrast, according to the men, was because the dads were ineligible for paid leave from their employer (which would be paid at their salary rate, rather than at the minimum wage).[17]

By 2024, 68 per cent of Australian private employers with at least 100 staff offered paid parental leave. However, men made up only 17 per cent of those who took that leave as their child's primary carer.[18] A quarter of employers said they had a target to lift the number of men taking parental leave.[19]

In the book *At a Turning Point*, Professor Marian Baird and Emeritus Professor Gillian Whitehouse argue the taxpayer-funded system has lacked incentives for fathers to 'share the care' and 'does not challenge the highly gendered division of care responsibilities between women and men in Australia'.[20] From 2026, four weeks out of the 26-week allocation is reserved for each parent in a couple on a 'use it or lose it' basis. An explainer on the Department of Social Services website says 'this will help to encourage greater sharing of care responsibilities' but there are concerns the changes don't go far enough to really shift the dial.[21] Professor Baird, who was involved in evaluations that led to the reforms, argues the changes most likely to alter dads' behaviour would be to quarantine even more time for fathers and to pay that leave at a 'high-income replacement level', rather than the minimum wage. This could be done by government or by employers topping up the public scheme. 'It's a well-established pattern that in households where men earn more, they will continue to work,' Professor Baird told me. 'Most partners still seem to think when it comes to the crunch if someone has to take the time off it should be the mother.' (Anecdotally, women tell me this is also the case with employers who still seem surprised when the father in the family calls in sick, or asks about flex-time, rather than the mother.)

Currently, men who take parental leave usually take it straight after a baby is born, to be home to support the mother or older children. But they are not necessarily motivated by being there to care for the infant, Professor Baird said. 'The research is pretty strongly saying that unless fathers take leave by themselves and do the caring solo it won't actually change their caring behaviours later in life. We can't wait for fathers to come around to thinking, "I want to look after the baby." You have to put the policy in place first and that will change behaviours.'

There is international evidence to back this up. A US study of 10,000 children born in 2001 found dads who took longer parental leave after a birth were more involved in child care nine months later.[22] Other analysis of working fathers in Australia, Denmark, the UK and the US found dads who take at least two weeks' parental leave are more likely to do tasks like changing nappies, feeding children, giving baths, reading books and waking at night for a child.[23]

Adelaide dad Arman, who we met earlier, is among the minority of fathers to take extended time off paid work to parent. During six months' unpaid leave from his then role in the South Australian public service he got 'a bit of a rude shock', finding the daily parenting responsibilities were 'never-ending'. As a particularly social and busy person, the most frustrating aspect for Arman was that he 'wasn't able to do anything'. Anyone who has spent time caring for young children will know what he means. It wasn't that Arman had no idea what he was in for. He has always been the chief nappy changer in their household, lain down with the kids while they fall asleep and sprung out of bed in the night to collect a baby for Genevieve to breastfeed. But without the 'break' of being with other adults and working without interruption, he came to fully understand the relentlessness of being the primary carer.

When their second son was born in 2023 the couple's financial situation had changed and they could only afford for Arman to take a month off work, using annual and unpaid leave. The contrast in experience led him to lobby the

South Australian government to extend paid parental leave entitlements to fathers or non-birthing parents in the public service. The government said in mid-2023 that it was 'actively considering' making leave provisions more flexible, but this had not happened by the time I finished writing this book. Nationally, change is afoot though, with the first review of maternity leave provisions for federal public servants since 1973 recommending an increase from 12 to 18 weeks' paid leave and that the leave be extended to biological or adoptive parents, of any gender.[24]

As we know, full-time stay-at-home dads are pretty rare in Australia. An estimate from 2016, based on ABS data, suggests there were about 75,000 of them, compared with about 500,000 stay-at-home-mums.[25] Australian Institute of Family Studies researcher Jennifer Baxter has found children in stay-at-home father families tend to be older and mothers 'still take on much of the caring and household work even if fathers have increased responsibility for child care'. It is 'uncommon' for fathers to 'always or usually' do key parenting tasks, she notes. Or, in other words, to be the default.

Baxter analysed data from the Household, Income and Labour Dynamics in Australia (HILDA) Survey between 2002 and 2015, involving families where at least one parent was employed. Out of six categories of child-care tasks (dressing, playing, helping with homework, transport, bedtime routine and staying home with sick kids), *only one* was done solely by dads more often than mums. In many cases dads were the main parent doing a particular task less than 10 per cent of the time. This was regardless of whether it was mum staying home or dad, *or* a home where both parents worked.[26]

I quoted her early in this book but it is worth repeating: Baxter's research has shown, simply, that 'children were at all times more likely to be with their mother than their father'. Is this not the definition of default parent? Baxter broke down every minute of the day that four- and five-year-old children spent with their parents and the numbers make it clear: on weekdays the children spent 406 minutes with mum and 182 with dad. (The rest at school, extra-curricular activities or with other carers etc.) On weekends children spent 500 minutes with mum and 402 with dad, *but* the time they spent with their father 'very often overlapped with the time they spent with their mother', Baxter found.[27]

The above is not intended to paint dads as lazy or indifferent, but to illustrate that fatherhood does not seem to markedly change men's lives in the same way, or with the same uniformity, as motherhood changes women's.

For most Aussie kids, the default setting is mum. Admittedly this can be a privilege; we get to be their first choice, their favourite person, their safe place. But it can also be draining, or enraging. And it can be rough on the dads who want to be more involved but instead cop some version of 'Not you!' on a daily or nightly basis.

It's not usually dad's fault if the kids prefer mum, but the tension caused by an obvious default can make parenting as a team pretty tricky. Some of my meltdowns have come purely from seeing how differently (read: quietly and cooperatively) our kids behave for their father, but the minute I emerge its madness. It can be hard not to take this out on the only other adult in the room and that can cause big problems for the state of the union.

Who said it would be 50/50?

Parenting is rough on relationships. The strongest bonds are tested and if there are cracks beforehand, a baby will jackhammer them wide open. Even one of the world's most high-profile and successful mothers, former US First Lady Michelle Obama, has conceded that her relationship with husband and former president Barack hit the skids after daughters Malia and Sasha came along, in 1998 and 2001. In an interview with Oprah Winfrey in the 2023 Netflix special *The Light We Carry* Obama laughed as she recalled how their daughters 'ruined all the love ... with their cuteness and their needing to eat all the time and their inability to communicate. And you can't be mad at them ...' So, who else could she direct her irritation at? 'Oh, it's you, it's your fault, Barack Obama,' she exclaimed. In an admission that was particularly comforting to me, the woman who popularised taking the high road in arguments (literally – remember 'When they go low, we go high'?) acknowledged that she could be 'hot-headed' and not always calmed by reason.[1]

New parenthood is a perilous time for couples. A 2019 survey of 2000 British mums and dads by ChannelMum and The Baby Show found one in five couples broke up in the year after having a child.[2] A third said their sex life evaporated and a quarter had no time for each other. Another quarter said when they did spend time together, all they did was argue. Other research has found having multiple children in quick succession is associated with an increased risk of separation. Couples in Finland who had a second child within 18 months of the first were between 24 and 49 per cent more likely to be divorced after ten years, compared with couples who waited up to four years between kids – regardless of age or socioeconomic status.[3] (As a mother of siblings born 20 months apart, I found reading this both alarming and validating!)

After lack of sleep, the most common factors contributing to overall levels of rage among the Angry Mums Club were inequality in the parenting load and the demands of running a house. Of 200 mums, 110 ticked each box. The household workload increases dramatically but, as we've learned, the majority of that extra burden is (*still*) usually worn by mum. You could pick from any number of datasets to make this argument, but let's look at the long-running HILDA Survey again. In 2019, HILDA tells us, Australian women *without* kids were doing an average 48.5 hours of paid and unpaid work while their childless male counterparts were putting in 46.3 hours. In contrast, mums and dads were both working at least 27 hours *more* each week – whether they were paid for it or not. And more often than not, mum isn't getting paid. As we learned in Part One, in 2019, each week mothers were doing almost 21 hours more unpaid work – like cleaning, cooking and child care – than fathers. That gap has shrunk from almost 29 hours back in 2002. Interestingly, HILDA says this isn't so much because dads have picked up the slack (doing about three hours more) as because mums, it seems, are actively resisting. We've cut almost five hours from our unpaid to-do list.[4] As I read this, I wondered whether houses were just messier or if we're outsourcing more of that previously unpaid work to paid cleaners and child carers or supermarket convenience meals. Either way, Aussie mums are still doing an average of almost seven hours of unpaid work *every day*, compared with dads' almost four hours. You might think single mums have it even worse, given they have no partner to try to share the load with. But HILDA looked at their schedules too and found they were doing a few hours *less* unpaid work a week than partnered mums. (Apparently, estimates for single fathers are unreliable 'due to small sample sizes'.)

When we look at how this division of unpaid labour pans out as our children grow, the numbers are the kind that make you want to laugh so you don't cry (or scream). In 2019, for parents with children aged six or younger, mum is doing almost double the unpaid work of dad (almost 61 hours compared to about 31.5 hours a week). The gap closes to about 11 hours when kids hit puberty. At no age or stage of their child's development is dad doing more than mum. And HILDA points out that between the first decade of this century and the second there has been 'almost no discernible change in these patterns'.[5]

And the differences start from day one. AIFS researcher Jennifer Baxter has tracked how many hours mums and dads spend each week on paid work, childcare and housework from the birth of their first child.[6]

Let's start with child care. Based on data from 2019, both mum and dad start at zero for hours spent parenting. In the first few months after baby arrives, dad's parenting hours rise to about 18 a week, but by the time bubs is three years old dad's hours begin to drop, eventually settling around eight a week – or just over an hour a day – by the time the kid is 12. In contrast, mum's parenting hours rocket straight up to more than 45 each week with an infant. Because she's had such a steep rise, she also has a steeper fall as the baby becomes a slightly less reliant toddler and an even more independent preschooler. But it takes until the kid is nine years old for her hours to drop down to dad's peak! By the time the kid is 12, mum's still doing about four or five hours more parenting per week than dad.

Looking at paid employment, dad's hours barely waver over the 12 years from his starting point of an (arguably high) 46-hour work week. But mum's plummet from around 34 hours down to an average of eight after bubs arrives, climbing back up to about 20 hours when the kid is ready for school. By the time they hit high school, mum is averaging about 28 hours of paid work.

And, finally, if that doesn't make you ragey enough, have a look at how much housework they're doing. Dad starts out doing around 15 hours a week and basically stays there, rising marginally to about 18 hours by the time the kid is on the edge of teenagehood. Mum's hours surge the minute bubs is born, doubling from the same 15 hours dad was doing to 30 hours, and basically staying put for evermore.

Domestic duties have been one of my toughest ongoing mum rage triggers. As the kids get older I'm getting more sleep, but the amount of cleaning and feeding has only grown, as have my hours of paid work. Admittedly, I've never loved housework (just ask my parents). I used to feel a lot better about it when my partner and I would divide and conquer on a Saturday morning, record player blaring, and it was all done in a couple of hours before we headed off for brunch. Out of mind until the next weekend rolled around. But now the four-person household to-do list feels never-ending. (Again, I wonder how mums of many do it.) My partner is definitely more houseproud than me. He'll get out the vacuum cleaner if there are a few toast crumbs or grains of sand on the floor. He mows the lawn, cleans the showers, remembers to put the bins out, changes the dead batteries and is definitely the one we want packing the car for a family holiday. If he makes a big pancake breakfast, he'll handwash all the bowls and frypans. I have to drag myself to do these kinds of things, and I can definitely hold out longer in a competition to see who can look at a sink overflowing with dirty crockery the longest before caving and running the tap. But, while the kids are young and I have either been on maternity leave or working part-time, I have been home for more hours on more days so simple mathematics means I have had to deal with more mess, more often. And cleaning this mess is the kind of work that is constant. Unlike the hero jobs of making a Sunday roast (a special skill of my partner's) or mowing the lawn once a fortnight, there is none of the satisfaction of pausing to admire my handiwork, knowing it will be some time before I have to repeat the task. Having washed enough clothes to see the bottom of the empty wash basket, I turn around to see all the clean clothes piled on one of the kids' beds, waiting to be put away. There is always another snack to be prepared and more food to be collected from the supermarket.

Managing my mum rage over housework has involved automating (I do a big clean on Mondays so I don't have to think about the toilets or mopping again for a week), asking for help (the grandparents take at least one of the kids so I can knock it out while listening to a podcast), actively resisting (other people's expectations of how often or thoroughly I should clean, including my partner's) and axing the guilt (the house is liveable, it's good enough).

In mother of two Nicky's case, a glaring lack of support and equality at home was one of the core issues that she feels led to the breakdown of her marriage – but she had to go through some extreme experiences to realise it. Nicky breezed through her first pregnancy but, on reflection, was unprepared for what was coming. Within months of giving birth she was admitted to a mother–baby unit following a diagnosis of postpartum depression and psychosis. It began as feeling exhausted and frustrated, then increasingly anxious, isolated and angry.

The anger was probably a warning sign, Nicky told me when we spoke years later. But things had to get a whole lot worse before she got the help she needed. When her son was a few months old she began having paranoid thoughts, including that she was going to die. 'I experienced a lot of guilt too, as I became more unwell.' She tried visiting a few different GPs but didn't feel they took her distress seriously. One mentioned postpartum depression but there was no follow-up. Eventually, things got so bad that Nicky's then husband took her to the emergency department. She was admitted to a psychiatric ward, where she was separated from her baby for a week until a bed opened up at a public mother–baby unit. By this point Nicky had stopped eating and drinking and was convinced she was on borrowed time. Inside the facility she tried medication, talk therapy and electroconvulsive therapy (ECT).

When we sat together in Nicky's living room while her two kids were at school, she told me she now believed that a lack of support 'was the trigger for my postnatal depression. I just sank because of the rage. It took down my mental health because I had these expectations [of support] ... and the frustration I had with feeling like I was someone that wasn't in a respectful and caring relationship. If you're living with constant disrespect and lack of empathy, then that [anger] scale can flip off the chart.'

I asked her if she can remember the first time her mum rage erupted. It prompted her to reflect, with fresh eyes, on the day the couple left hospital with their first child. 'His job was to fit the car capsule. When we got to the car he didn't know how to put it in properly, so we had to ask another man in the car park.' They set off for home and she was 'really angry and really rude. I just felt this irrational anger.' After doing the hard work of bringing their baby safely into the world, Nicky felt her partner had let the side down.

Quite often, when mums finally reveal that we are not coping, the response will come: 'Why didn't you ask for help?' Nicky *did* ask 'all the time' but said help rarely came. 'I'd be telling him I need help, this is really hard, or I can't change another diaper, and he's not listening.' When the couple eventually separated, she felt 'a lot happier and a lot calmer. I was a lot busier, and it was really hard but ... I have very defined boundaries now. I'm a different person. I've learned that in certain situations you just have to be really assertive, and that might sometimes be interpreted as rude, especially by people who have walked all over your boundaries in the past.'

I've said repeatedly that one of the keys to getting on top of my mum rage was learning to ask for support. Thankfully, once I got over my own awkwardness and guilt, I usually had a good response. But Nicky has touched on something really important. When our requests fall on deaf ears it can be rage-inducing.

Louisa, the mum in her late 30s who we met in Part Two, told me she experiences this to the point where she second-guesses herself. 'Am I being too passive? Am I not saying it clearly enough? What am I doing wrong?' she asked as we chatted over coffee at a suburban pub. Perhaps most infuriating, though, is the use of 'weaponised incompetence'.[7] Also known as 'strategic incompetence', this tactic can be employed by partners and serves to make it so difficult to outsource or handball even the simplest of tasks that mums end up feeling it is just easier to do it themselves. Note that we're not talking about gatekeeping here, where mum may unreasonably want something done a certain way, which pushes a willing dad out. Here, the deployer of this tactic wants mum to step in, so they can step out. 'It's infuriating,' Louisa said, adding that one of the worst battle grounds in her home was the laundry. 'I refuse to wash his clothes,' she said of her husband, and I mentally congratulated her for actively resisting. 'It's enough that I wash, hang out, fold and put away mine and the kids' laundry. But the only thing I've asked is, if he's undressing them for the bath or bed, to turn the kids' clothes the right way around if they are inside out.

Otherwise, the dirt from food and the school playground doesn't come off in the washing machine. I'm not sure how many times I have asked him to do this, but he just won't do it ... so I just do it myself.'

Asking for help outside the immediate family unit can also backfire. Louisa, who is also a foster carer, gave me a few examples, like the time she was in a last-minute bind and asked a relative to look after one of her kids – because this relative had offered to be an emergency option – only to be knocked back. Or the time she asked a foster care agency to fund a cleaning service because she had been sick, on top of managing ongoing chronic conditions. 'I said, "I'm struggling, I can't keep up,"' when the agency worker asked how they could help. But 18 months later, the cleaning service had still not been organised. Apparently, Louisa needed to provide proof that her conditions were impeding her ability to keep her house clean. 'I don't have time for that because I have to keep this house clean, and my body and my brain are not coping,' she said, exasperated. 'So even when you ask for help, you feel guilty about it, and you feel angry because you're desperately trying to get help and no one listens.'

Anger in mothers has been recognised as a cry for help – rather than a personality flaw – in two studies we've already touched on. In their analysis of 278 sleep-deprived Canadian mothers, researchers noted that women may 'resort' to anger when the expressing of other emotions such as sadness or anxiety 'fails to elicit sufficient support'.[8] It was similarly explained in the 'Seeing red' paper, whose authors noted that displays of anger by mums served to call attention to their 'distress over violated expectations and compromised needs'.

Disheartingly, this wasn't always received helpfully by others, and the mums instead became 'angry at themselves' for perceived failures.[9]

Asking for help is hard. Often the response to an admission of struggle is encouragement. 'You've got this,' they tell us. But when we feel like we don't 'got' it, when that vulnerability is dismissed or diminished, it can be crushing. Sociologist Dr Sophie Brock agreed when I put this to her. 'It's not enough to say, "Oh yes, we see all the pressures that mothers are under so we totally understand why they're angry,"' she said. 'On one hand we say, "You're supermum, you can do it all" ... then on the other hand we actually don't show up when she says that she doesn't want to be supermum, she just wants help.'

Dude, where's my village?

It takes a village to raise a kid, they tell us, but not all villages are created equal. Some are a thriving metropolis. Others are like the set of a bad Western, tumbleweeds rolling down the main street. In my village live two sets of willing, able and trustworthy grandparents, a team of paid child carers, a collection of aunties, uncles, cousins and stand-in grandparents with a little time to spare, and a diverse circle of mum and dad friends in the trenches with us. And I still meltdown!

Almost everyone I interviewed for this book mentioned 'the village' at one point or another. Almost half the Angry Mums Club identified a sparse or non-existent village as contributing to their anger in motherhood, and a third felt lonely or isolated. The general consensus is that a supportive village is still the solution to many of our problems … but it is also becoming an endangered species. The village used to be inside our home, with multiple generations of the same family living under one roof. It used to be in our street, when we knew and trusted our neighbours and would let our kids play outside. It used to be in the best friends we could call night or day. But what happens when everyone in the village already has their hands full? If all your friends or siblings have kids around the same time, you all know exactly what support the others need but are too busy to give it. The rising cost of living and expectations of intensive mothering mean everyone is so caught up working and getting to school and swimming lessons and trying to prepare meals and get some sleep that arranging to spend time with other families requires the planning of a military operation. Just dropping in to check on someone is unheard of.

When I was young, I spent a *lot* of time at my second home – my best friend's house. She's the closest thing I have to a sister and we would spend alternate weekends at each other's house. At her place, we would swim in the backyard pool and play an absurdly long-running game of Monopoly while we ate big bowls of homemade soup. At my house, we'd go to the beach and then come home to eat muffins my mum baked and play with our original Cabbage Patch dolls. (I know I'm really ageing myself there.)

Little did we know these play dates weren't just for our benefit. Each week, when one of us would wave goodbye and scuttle inside our friend's house, our mother would get back in the car, sigh with relief, and drive home to spend the rest of the weekend holed up in her office writing. Our families met because our mums worked at the same university, and my friend and I attended the onsite childcare. The story goes that at our first meeting I threw sand at her in the sandpit, but she has somehow seen fit to put up with me for the next three and a half decades. I'm now a godmother to three of her kids, and her parents spoil my two like another set of grandparents.

Also in my childhood village were primary school friends who lived a few houses away and had older siblings. We would ride our bikes home from school and stay at one another's house until our parents got home from work. On other days, I went to after-school care, which remains a lifeline for many working parents.

Looking back, it all seemed to work quite well. But as a mum I now understand that finding people you trust to look after your child, with whom your child wants to spend time, and with whom you can coordinate schedules, cannot be taken for granted. Not everyone can attend school close to home and make friends with the neighbours. It can be hard to forge a strong connection with other parents from childcare, kindergarten or school through a few minutes of small talk at drop-off. And at some schools it is impossible to secure a place in after-school care, or you must join a waitlist and hope for the best. A national teacher shortage post Covid means educators can take their pick of better paid classroom jobs and there are fewer willing to work for lower pay in out-of-school-hours care (OSHC) or vacation care. Given this is the only option for many families, governments are trying to make OSHC more accessible by broadening the range of qualifications workers can hold. The logistical juggle is even worse if you're trying to send your kid to public preschool, where hours are even less compatible with a nine-to-five workday. Only select preschools in New South Wales and Victoria offer after-hours care. In South Australia a trial at kindergartens has begun to encourage more working families to take advantage of the early education.

The Covid lockdowns in the early 2020s highlighted the need for a village while simultaneously cutting us off from many parts of it. Expecting and new parents reported frustration with being disconnected from their support network, without any choice or control. The timing felt unfair and they described that period as 'horrible', 'stressful', 'anxious' and 'exhausting'.[1] Our first child was born just as the pandemic was spreading overseas. As luck would have it, my neighbour was also pregnant and our daughters were born just a few months apart. In the absence of the cancelled mothers' group meet-ups, we passed long afternoons with cranky babies by walking to a nearby park where we would sit far apart on picnic rugs. Other days we chatted over the back fence, and when a snap lockdown ruined plans for my daughter's first birthday the neighbours celebrated with us outside on our adjoining driveways. It was comforting in those uncertain, early days of parenthood – and the pandemic – to know we weren't alone.

Around the same time, as if she knew isolated mums would be needing all the help they could get, mother-of-two Dinah Thomasset launched Villagehood Australia. Since then, the charity has helped more than 2000 mothers and children through coffee meetings, group sessions, education and safety in numbers. I met Dinah when I interviewed her for *The Advertiser* newspaper about her downward spiral into postnatal depression and how it sparked the idea for Villagehood Australia. At her lowest point, a chronically sleep-deprived Dinah remembers lying on her bathroom floor thinking, 'I don't want to be here.' Two days later she was hospitalised with severe pain. Blood tests suggested the alarming potential diagnosis of liver cancer, but when a doctor later told her that the situation was not life-threatening Dinah had a lightbulb moment. 'The idea that I might die stopped me from wanting to die,' she told me of that moment in late 2018. 'I realised all the expectations I was putting on myself were too much. Loving my children was enough. That changed everything for me.' After Dinah was released from hospital her GP referred her to a psychologist and she was diagnosed with postnatal depression. She and her husband sought help from a sleep consultant and Dinah took a trip to her birth country, Morocco, where she 'cried and cried and cried with my mum'. Being back with her 'village' – including eight aunties – made Dinah realise 'we're not meant to be doing this [parenting] alone'.

Today, women who come through Villagehood Australia say they feel 'a sense of relief ... We're opening a door to them so they can come be with their children, not having to worry about the way they look, and just show up,' Dinah told me. 'There are toys for the kids, volunteers to help. We always provide fruit and some yummy cake. They are talking to other women ... connected to a community. We are filling their cup.' For many mothers it is also about readjusting their perception of themselves as they go through the upheaval of matrescence. 'You may be respected in your career, you're highly skilled and people look up to you, and then you become a mother and they don't even look at you anymore,' Dinah said. These women tell her, 'I had a high status in my community, in my work, and now I'm here changing poops.' And that's what can spark the fury.

After a while Dinah started offering the Mummy Chat program, which takes mums through an eight-week course in a small group. It is there, in those more intimate and supported conversations, that they open up 'about their moment of anger, or resentment or frustration'.

The Reily Foundation CEO Nadia Bergineti told me that many of the parents she works with – who have had children removed by authorities – don't have 'anyone who could come and take them for a coffee or just say, "You have a nap and I will look after the baby."' The majority of families who come through the foundation's doors 'would be completely isolated', she said. 'They haven't necessarily had childcare, [because] there has been financial insecurity. They've got no friends to be able to debrief with. There is no respite.' Without family or social networks, and when they are 'feeling heightened constantly' by stress or trauma, it is difficult to regulate their emotions 'because you never get a minute of peace'. In some cases, this can be the trigger for turning to alcohol or other substances to self-medicate or mask uncomfortable feelings, 'because there's no one there to step in and just take the kids or have the conversation'. The internet jokes about 'mummy wine culture' but the habit of reaching for the bottle every evening once the kids are in bed is, in many cases, a coping mechanism. It's not ideal or recommended, but overwhelmed, under-resourced mothers are grasping for something they can do to quieten the mental load or ease stress and anxiety – without leaving home – that is cheaper and more easily available than therapy or babysitting.

When I spoke to Bergineti, an Italian mother of three from a large extended family, she reflected on the contrast between her clients and her own experience. 'I've struggled to go to my own husband and say, "I'm not coping today." I've had an anger with myself that I couldn't do things properly,' she said of her early motherhood. 'But I had that village around me that could step in and identify that the washing was getting out of control and just put a load on for me. Back in the day, in Italy, there would be a village, a community. We put too much pressure on ourselves now to be and do everything.'

Sometimes, for me, the only thing that can help reset the rage is a proper break. I'm not talking an hour while the kids watch TV. I'm talking a string of hours when they are physically away from me and my mind can switch off, without worrying about them. This was extremely difficult for me at first. I didn't spend a night away from either of my children until they were both almost one. It wasn't until my kids were four and two that I spent two whole nights without them (amid a not-insignificant amount of guilt). When I came to pick them up from my parents' house late on a Sunday morning, my dad answered the door and told me I looked like I'd been on a holiday. It was staggering what a difference it made to be able to sleep through the night, two nights in a row, and wake up at 7 am instead of 5 am. I even worked my paid job on Saturday and still felt rested. (Mum and Dad on the other hand needed a good lie down!)

A survey of more than 2300 grandparents of children aged under 13 (overwhelmingly grandmothers) in mid-2021, by the Australian Institute of Family Studies (AIFS), found a quarter babysat at least once a week. One in five who provided regular care put in 20 or more hours a week. Many had retired or cut back their own work hours to do so, including one 62-year-old grandmother who was forgoing $380 a week to give 'expected' care to her grandkids. Another, also 62, couldn't babysit because she'd gone part-time while raising her own children and had to keep working in her 60s to accrue enough superannuation for her retirement.

Almost a quarter of grandparents who provided care said it was difficult to balance with other responsibilities. And some felt their child took advantage by asking for frequent care. Almost 30 per cent of nans and pops felt they couldn't say no. One granny, aged 61, said she 'no longer want[ed] the responsibility of caring for children'. Another, aged 72, resented that 'I only see them when help is needed'. In contrast, one 82-year-old nana told how she enjoyed spending time with her son and grand-daughter together. They would visit her to pass time while the mother worked. This too is a village. Having somewhere to go, someone to talk to who can distract your kids, provide a buffer or a change of scenery. Someone you can just pop in on.

The most common reason for recruiting grandparents as babysitters was so parents could do paid work, including when children were too sick to go to childcare or school. Most told the AIFS survey they were happy to do it. 'It's even better than having your own children because you are not so busy and so you have time to soak up the moments,' one grandma, 66, said.[2]

But relying on grandparents is not an option for everyone. Family estrangements, children with high-care needs, living interstate or overseas, and grandparent disability or chronic pain were among the reasons 40 per cent of grandies surveyed never provide care to grandchildren.[3] In other cases, grandparents may still be working, be ageing, unwell or immuno-compromised, or have passed away. Or the relationship may not be a trusted one. In my chats with a group of experienced social workers I was reminded that a lot of mums who have grown up in the child protection system, or under its surveillance, can't rely on their parents because they weren't safe guardians in their own childhoods. Mental illness, family violence or drug and alcohol abuse may mean large portions of the wider family – siblings, aunts, uncles – aren't safe or able to look after children either. Or they may have had family ties severed by being taken into care and have not been able to repair or reconnect. These same life circumstances may mean that mum doesn't have the financial resources, or meet the criteria, to use paid childcare. Let alone that her history of trauma may make it even harder to trust strangers to look after her children.

This is particularly relevant for First Nations mothers, who live with the intergenerational trauma of colonisation, shorter life expectancies and persistently higher rates of removal of their children into state care. One Aboriginal mother told me her children 'did not go anywhere' because of the fear they would be judged, reported or removed. For her, the village is her extended, but close, family. Large sibling groups mean plenty of hands to help change babies, make bottles and cuddle little ones to sleep. Mirning and Kokatha mum of three April Lawrie said the concept of the village, or mob, is 'part of our cultural practice. We have a large notion of family. Nanas and aunties, they will growl you [tell you off] if you growl your kids. They will pull you into line because that's grandmother's lore in Aboriginal culture.' But it cannot be taken for granted that all Aboriginal mothers have that village. Lawrie said many have had to move from Country to cities to study, work or find housing and are physically separated from their support network. The higher rates of removal of Aboriginal children into state care are also 'severing ties' between thousands of young Aboriginal mums- and dads-to-be and their mob. Lawrie said part of the solution lies in investment in more Aboriginal-run community programs 'led by Aboriginal women for Aboriginal women ... That's where you get your help, because you're not popping your head up to the people who don't understand you. It's about cultural safety. It's about trusting and knowing that you're with people that aren't going to judge you and are there to help you.'

Sitting around a long dining table with the group of senior social workers I consulted for this book, I asked if there was a place where a mother who's not coping can go for free, non-judgemental help, where the staff or volunteers won't be likely, or obligated, to make a report about her. There was a lengthy silence. They looked around the table at one another. Not much came to mind. There are places like Villagehood Australia, but the scarcity of options is just more evidence that our society is set up to surveil, rather than support, struggling mums.

Women who don't have anyone to watch their children, or anywhere else to send them, just have to take the kids with them everywhere. I heard of one mother who had to take her four children to her dentist appointment but when she arrived was told that the kids couldn't be in the treatment room. So she was unable to get dental care. Imagine how furious you would be, having found time for the appointment and got four children there, only to find out that you wouldn't be treated. Then having to get them all home again – and reschedule the appointment.

Sometimes the only option for respite is to pay for it. Like the $50 I parted ways with on a particularly challenging solo-parenting Saturday to cover entry to an indoor playground and two kids' meals. In return, I got four hours of relatively hands-off parenting and time to drink a hot coffee on my own. It's more likely, though, that we're paying for childcare, which can certainly be part of the village. I have been exceptionally grateful to the women and men who have kept our children safe and happy while their father and I worked. And even more so on days when I was struggling with an endo flare-up and I could drop the kids at childcare or preschool and go home for a sick day. But childcare can be an expensive respite option. KindiCare data reported in 2024 showed the nation's most expensive centre, in New South Wales, charged $210.42 a day and the cheapest, in Tasmania, charged $148.13.[4] Other analysis by iSelect using data from the ABS and Education Department found families in many parts of Australia are spending 40 per cent of their household income (or more) on childcare fees.[5]

The Australian government offers a Child Care Subsidy (CCS) that reduces the out-of-pocket cost for eligible families, but it is a complicated system. Put as simply as possible, for eligible families the federal government pays the childcare provider a proportion of the daily fee and parents pay the gap. The CCS is means-tested based on a family's income, and parents have been made to pass an activity test by proving how many hours they are working, looking for work, studying or volunteering each week. Parents who earn more pay more of a gap, on a sliding scale. The government puts a cap on the amount it will cover, which is intended to dissuade centres from fleecing the taxpayer (given the system already costs $15 billion a year).[6] It doesn't appear to have worked, though, as about a third of centres charge over the hourly rate cap, raising out-of-pocket costs for parents.[7]

In 2024 the Productivity Commission released a long-awaited examination of Australia's childcare system, which urged reforms to make it more accessible, affordable and inclusive. Among the recommendations was scrapping the activity test (proving how many hours a parent works), which it argued was confusing and 'does little to incentivise labour force participation'. It also gives some parents the impression that childcare is 'only for people who have jobs' and puts them off seeking support.[8] In early 2025 the federal government introduced laws to scrap the test, and guarantee three days of subsidised early education from 2026 for every child in a family earning less than $530,000 a year. Government modelling has estimated this change will help about 66,700 families.[9]

More than one in five Australian children are developmentally behind their peers in at least one area by the time they start school[10] and there are more than 100,000 kids aged five or younger on the National Disability Insurance Scheme (NDIS).[11] For their families, finding suitable and affordable childcare can be incredibly difficult, time-consuming and frustrating. The Association for Children with Disability has reported that families encounter a range of 'tactics' used by childcare operators to deny them access, including 'making it clear their child is not welcome', telling them that the childcare centre does not have the funding or staff to support their child, and restricting how many hours their child can attend.[12] That would piss off any mum, or dad.

The Australian government funds the Inclusion Support Program to enable mainstream childcare centres to hire extra, specialised staff to work with children with high needs. In 2024–25 it was allocated $230 million but the Productivity Commission found this is not meeting demand, which 'has been increasing rapidly'.[13] This is something mum Etta knows all too well. Having to fight for her son to be included is a major source of rage for her. She and her husband Oliver knew that their third child, William, would need surgery for a heart condition after he was born. They didn't know he would also be born blind and go on to be diagnosed with epilepsy at age four and an intellectual disability at age seven. Now ten, William has the developmental capacity of a four-year-old and needs support with toileting, washing, dressing, eating and taking his medication. Etta, 44, also has two daughters, Tilly and Sara, 15 and 12, who had to 'grow up really quickly' while her focus was on keeping their brother alive. 'There was so much they missed out on,' she told me when we met at a playground with her family. 'I was acutely aware of it as it was going along but you can't do anything about it.'

At one point Etta was managing three kids under the age of five, largely alone, in the country town where they lived. Oliver was working full-time, Etta's parents had passed away and her siblings were living interstate. 'We were alone,' she explained. 'I was sad, upset and angry that I had been dealt another difficult card on top of losing both my parents. I resented having William at times and remember thinking that he had "ruined" my life. It made me angry and very lonely. I would snap at the kids because our life wasn't the same as it had been before William.'

Instead, life was full of medical appointments, paperwork, worry and fear. At five months old, William had to be collected in an ambulance, unconscious, after contracting a virus. At six months, he underwent open-heart surgery. He gained some vision as he grew but his brain has difficulty computing the images his eyes take in. He can't be left alone to eat. The family has never been to the cinema together and a 'quick trip to the shops' is unheard of. 'To take William to the grocery store took four years of occupational therapy ... teaching him skills to safely get out of the car or hold my hand in the car park,' Etta explained. 'Otherwise, it was too overwhelming so he would just run.'

William is cheeky, sweet and full of energy. He loves to draw, swim in the backyard pool, play tackle with Tilly and Sara, or sit at the dining table for a card game. The girls help with day-to-day care and keeping their brother entertained, but every day is a marathon for Etta. 'To wake up, get ready, eat breakfast, leave the house, a simple trip would take all of my energy,' she said. 'Not many people understand. To get support meant paying money. But to have William looked after meant more money, because of his needs.'

William has been on the NDIS since birth, for services including occupational therapy, speech therapy and physiotherapy, but Etta had to fight for approval to hire a support worker. Now there is someone to take William to and from the special school he joined after Etta felt he was pushed out of mainstream education. She told me she'd had to advocate every term for adequate funding and was constantly asked by teachers how to deal with William.

Mothering a child with special needs shrank Etta's potential village because, she believed, 'people didn't know how to support me'. She and William weren't invited to play dates because William was unpredictable. If they were invited, they often couldn't go because he needed to be home for a sleep – something other children his age had grown out of. Etta opened up to her GP one day and was prescribed antipsychotic medication, 'which just made me even angrier ... I just needed support, a break, some sleep, someone to drop off a meal, someone to bathe my kids and put them to bed or the ability to go for a walk by myself.'

In the absence of a village of family or friends, Etta would have benefited so much from the support of skilled and affordable child carers. William was enrolled at the same centre as his sisters for a while and the staff were kind, she said, but 'they didn't know how to support him. He would go right up to other kids' faces, or touch them, because of his low vision. I remember one mum saying to me, "What's wrong with him, why does he do that?" Even when I explained, she looked at me as if to say, "Make him stop."'

The argument for investing more taxpayer funds into services like childcare is usually made on the economic basis of getting more people into work. But what about the mums with no other type of village? The mums like Etta who need respite from caring 24/7 for children with high needs. The mums who are home with their children because they can't job search with toddlers in tow. Or the mums who need someone to step in so they can take care of themselves before things get too bad – and no one in the village is answering their phone. Like the woman who told the Productivity Commission how having access to paid childcare had enabled her to seek treatment for anxiety and postnatal depression. 'I was able to send my kids to DC [daycare] and know that they are loved, having fun and getting the attention they need while I was able to work on my issues,' she said.[14]

While the picture I've painted in the past few chapters could leave us all feeling a bit despondent at the pace of change, there are reasons to be optimistic. The scrapping of the childcare activity test is just one shift that will make a big difference for a lot of families, and will have longer-term ripple effects as the children who benefit from it become parents themselves. We will also start to see the impact of paying superannuation on parental leave and policy changes to encourage greater sharing of that paid leave by caregivers. Hopefully dads will take more advantage of flexible work options, and the gender pay gap will continue to inch closed. Until then we'll just have to keep relying on whatever patchwork of grandparents, neighbours or favours gets us through.

Dad's right of reply

By this point we're pretty clear on what it's like to be an angry mum. But what is it like to live with one? The time has come to get the perspective of the long-suffering and (usually) more even-tempered father of my children. He has borne the brunt of countless meltdowns – and been the cause of plenty too. When I decided to write this book, I promised him a right of reply. So one night we sent the kids off to the grandparents', opened a bottle of red wine and pressed record on my phone's voice app.

'So what's it like to live with a mum who is struggling to manage feelings of anger?' I asked him as we tucked into medium–rare steaks he had cooked on the barbecue.

'Frustrating,' was his first thought. A pause. Some chewing. Then: 'It often escalates from zero to a hundred very quickly. It's not an easy thing to be around. You've got to be on mental tippy toes.'

So far, I tended to agree. 'What do you think sets me off?' I prodded, and had to stifle the impulse to dispute what came next.

'Most of the time, I feel that the blow-ups come from your frustration with the kids, even if they're directed at me.'

I pushed a bit more and common ground emerged: lack of sleep, the kids behaving better for him than for me (that old default parent problem), stresses at work. Then he threw out a cheeky in-joke: 'It can be that someone didn't slice the cheese thin enough for you.'

Remember the story from my first Saturday back at work after maternity leave, receiving a phone call from my partner asking if our daughter could eat cheese? We actually have a bit of a history with cheese. Before kids, after I had my first surgery for endometriosis, my partner was looking after me and I asked him to make me a sandwich. When I saw him slicing the cheese for said sandwich I blew up, seemingly out of nowhere, because he was slicing it too thickly, at least for my taste. (Yep, I know ...) I was disproportionately upset because what his apparently cavalier attitude to the width of the cheese signalled to me, in my fragile state, was that he didn't care. I was coming off a general anaesthetic, my abdomen was sore and I was on some pretty strong painkillers – but it was, in hindsight, an overreaction. This little incident has since become a bit of a touchstone in our relationship for whether an argument is justified. The fact he has raised it in this conversation about my mum rage made me laugh, but I pressed on: 'You know it's not about the cheese, though, right?'

'I know it's not,' he conceded, but then he explained that it can be hard to know what *has* sparked the mum rage. 'I don't necessarily know what it is, the underlying thing that has set you off. Is it me, is it the kids, is it work, is it all of them? In those situations I can try and say something but anything will get construed in the wrong way.'

The cheese-slicing incident aside, when I asked him if he thought I was angry before we had kids, he agreed I was impatient and liked to be in control of things. Injustice or unfairness has always pissed me off and I have rarely been afraid to speak up for myself. I sometimes let my emotions get the better of me and gave people the odd serve on bad days. My partner and I absolutely fought pre-kids. But it's definitely different – and more frequent – now, he said. 'There might have been bits and pieces before, but kids just amplified it. This is not an easy time of life.'

In contrast, I would describe my partner as one of the most laid-back blokes I've ever met. Opposites must attract because I'm probably one of the most anxious overthinkers he knows. (We also barrack for rival AFL teams, but that's another story.) We are similar in many ways: our enjoyment of red wine, travel and home renovation shows, our core values and our hopes for the future. We both also *really* like to be right and to have things our way. A key difference, though, is how long we dwell on things. 'I have the ability to move on fairly quickly,' he said. 'A lot of things I will just let go eventually. It might be in that instance, or throughout the day or over a week, but there's not much that I will hold on to for a long period of time.'

'How?!' I blurted between mouthfuls of wine.

'At the end of the day I'm not as bothered by what other people think about me,' he replied. This, dear reader, is the clear-minded view of a man who has *not* internalised the rules of intensive mothering. As if to drive the point home, he went on: 'There's an ideal of parenting but I don't know one parent in the world who would have ever met it all the time.'

For the record, my partner does get angry. And he has done his share of yelling. 'I will raise my voice, quite loud and firm ... and I might need to walk away for a bit,' he admitted.

What sets him off? Usually, the kids being excessively loud, stubborn or not listening. Oh, and me telling him how to do stuff. 'If I started doing something with the kids and I have you come in and tell me how to do it a different way, or that I'm doing it wrong, you're second-guessing me. That would annoy me because then I think that you don't trust me. You're checking up on me.' Sometimes this has proven necessary, like when it is his week to make the school lunches and it gets to 8.15 am and the lunchbox is still sitting empty on the kitchen bench. Oftentimes, though, it can be the kind of gatekeeping I flagged earlier. The things mums can do, even unwittingly, that have the potential to push dads out. In the early days I did it through judgement about how my partner dressed our daughter, or if I felt he was holding her too carelessly or playing too riskily. I can still do it, about what he might let our kids watch on TV or eat for a treat or if we disagree about discipline. 'It has lessened,' he said, 'but it still happens.' He cites a recent example where I told him he had to change the dress pants he had put on our son for a day running around kicking a football. We have agreed to disagree about that one …

But when my partner loses his cool, does he end up in a guilt spiral like most of us angry mums?

'No, because there's no reason to,' he said matter-of-factly, causing me to almost spurt my shiraz. 'It's usually because I've told the kids something that they don't like, or they don't get what they want, so of course they're going to be upset. They always get what they need, but as a father I have to draw a line. Nothing's been done that is irreparable.' It's the same if his frustration is sparked by something I've done.

He'll let me know about it, but he doesn't harbour a grudge and he is much better at repairing without prompting.

He has a similar take on asking for help. While I have wrung my hands about recruiting grandparents in for a break, my partner says simply: 'I don't feel guilty about involving the grandparents in the children's lives. They cherish the time with them. It takes a village to raise a child, not just one person. I can do this on my own, but it'll be a lot easier if I don't have to.'

Indeed.

Epilogue: Am I still angry?

About halfway through writing this book, something happened that knocked me flat on my back. Not figuratively, but actually. Each night for about a week I had been collapsing into bed with a splitting headache the moment the kids were asleep. The pain had been getting progressively worse for weeks. Usually, by morning the headache would subside enough for me to take some paracetamol and ibuprofen and get back on the hamster wheel for another day, but by Sunday morning pushing through was no longer an option. My head felt like it was going to crack open and the resulting nausea was as bad as my persistent morning sickness had been.

You'll remember that in our household Sunday mornings are when my partner gets some kid-free time. So, this Sunday morning, I was standing in the kitchen around 7.30 am, head pounding, stomach gurgling and panic rising at the thought of corralling the kids for another few hours. After an hour of dressing, feeding and cleaning, they were settled on the couch watching *Play School* so I could finally eat breakfast. My partner was seated at our computer with a coffee, headphones on.

When I think back on what happened next, I can see just what a turning point this was. It is also the clearest example I can give of how I had internalised so many of the 'rules' of motherhood, how they contributed to my anger and why the tactics I now use to manage it are so important. (A reminder, they are: Awareness. Analysis. Asking for help. Automating. Actively resisting. Alone time. Axing the guilt.)

Back to my kitchen. By now, I was *aware* I wasn't going to be able to parent much at all that day, let alone solo. So I reached for my phone (and my village) and texted my mum to *ask* if she could help. She would have still been asleep, but just knowing back-up might be available soon made me feel a little better. Steadying myself against the kitchen bench, I began to *analyse* what I could do immediately to improve the situation. I had already *automated* child care by sticking the kids in front of the TV. I needed to take some stronger painkillers but couldn't until I'd eaten. I was also going to need to *ask* my partner for help. During the week I had been too tired and sore to properly explain to him how bad the headaches had been getting, so the interruption to his morning 'off' was going to come as a rude shock. Both of us look forward to those few weekend hours to ourselves and have both been guilty of letting an eye roll or exaggerated sigh give away our irritation if they are interrupted. Even though I was incapacitated by illness, through no fault of my own, I felt looming guilt at the prospect of cutting short what was supposed to be his *alone time*.

But there was no other way. *Axing that guilt* and *actively resisting* the expectation that I should soldier on, I tapped him on the shoulder. He half turned and pulled one earphone clear. 'Hey, I've got a really bad headache,' I said. 'I need to go upstairs to take some painkillers and lie down until they kick in. I know it's your morning, but I need you to watch the kids for a bit.' It tumbled out in a sheepish rush. He looked at me but didn't say anything. I went on: 'I've asked Mum, but I just need some help to get through until she can come round.' At this point, he went to say something about it being 'his' morning and that he was in the middle of something. 'I know,' I said, 'and I wouldn't ask unless I was really struggling.' We stared at each other. Aaaand then nothing. No move on his part to get up …

So I turned and slowly walked back to the kitchen. If I was going to have to grit this out, I needed to get some food in my stomach and take those painkillers. Then maybe I could just lie on the couch with the kids until the drugs kicked in. It wasn't until I reached the fridge that the rage hit me: *What about all the times I had brought him dinner or a cup of tea in bed when he was sick? All the times I'd put the kids to bed on my own so he could rest after a big day?* I'd been going through the motions of making myself a coffee and, all of a sudden, I slammed the microwave door. Then I started to cry. Hot tears of frustration and fury. Remember how we learned early on in this book that it's not just physical pain that spurs anger but having the pain ignored or feeling unsupported? This was that. I had summoned the courage to ask for help and I had been dismissed. I didn't want to upset the kids so I made a beeline for the stairs, as big audible sobs began escaping my mouth. I was so furious the waterworks were unstoppable. Upstairs I slammed our bedroom door and threw myself on the mattress.

After a minute, I heard my partner come in. He started to explain that he wasn't fobbing me off, he was still waking up and had wanted to finish something on the computer. Sure, he was a little irritated at having his limited window to himself cut short. But he now grasped how much I was struggling and he was sorry. Fair enough, but I was in no mood. I yelled at him to go away and eventually he did. When I returned downstairs ten minutes later, I wordlessly finished making my toast and coffee. I took the strong painkillers and eased onto the couch. The kids had been watching TV for over an hour by this point (cue more mum guilt), but I didn't have it in me to do anything except snuggle in next to them, close my eyes and give up. After a while, I heard some movement in the background. I opened an eye to see my partner packing a bag. He'd been in touch with Mum and she was coming around to take our daughter for the day. He was going to take our son to the playground. When they all left I went upstairs, crawled into bed and pulled the covers over my head.

Knowing everything I know now, I don't feel a scintilla of guilt when I look back on this meltdown. I know the anger I felt in that moment was signalling something was wrong and I had important needs that weren't being met. I was in pain, I was hungry, I felt burned out and was still somehow the default parent. It didn't come out of nowhere – the 'sequence of provocations' had been building for weeks as those headaches worsened (even if I hadn't communicated this very well) and I juggled paid work, housework and parenting. It wasn't until I was almost incapacitated that I had been able to override the rules I'd internalised about how the 'perfect' mum and partner would push through. When I finally asked for help and didn't get it, I was right to be angry. In the previous few years, even six months earlier, I would have felt guilt and shame for overreacting, for failing to control my emotions. But this time it felt different. For once, this was useful anger.

That one day in bed turned into a week, then another, and another. It turns out that years of breastfeeding in awkward positions, lugging children around, spending too much time working at a computer and holding all my stress as tension in my neck and jaw had finally caught up with me. I had to take some sick leave from work. My eyes hurt when I looked at anything bright. My fuse was short but it hurt to raise my voice even a little. I couldn't chase the kids if they ran away. I didn't have the energy to negotiate or argue. I felt like I was dragging myself through mud every day, counting the minutes until everyone was in bed. Having changed so much about my life to try to manage my mum rage, it felt like I'd been dropped right back in the worst of it.

Some days I thought I was starting to feel better – so I pushed it too far and ended up flat on my back again. Usually, this was because I was struggling to do nothing. I *should* have been working. I *should* have been writing. I *should* have been exercising, cleaning, cooking. I *should* have been doing something with the kids. But my body said no. I hadn't been listening to her for far too long and she was putting her foot down. As a result, I had more alone time than I knew what to do with and axing the guilt about that was hard. I didn't start to feel better until I accepted that I had to lower my expectations. So the kids watched more TV. Reading them books at bedtime was replaced with lying down next to their warm little bodies to listen to an audiobook. The grandparents stepped up their babysitting hours. We ate more takeaway. The house stayed messy. And our sweet girl and boy loved it. They would gently pat my shoulder, give me kisses and tell me they would look after me.

During the hours I spent lying down, staring at my bedroom ceiling, I thought about all the mums soldiering on through chronic fatigue, cancer treatment, dialysis, persistent pain, severe morning sickness or grief. A large part of me felt embarrassed for being so impaired by something I believed I'd brought upon myself. *If I just had better posture. If I wasn't such a stress head.* But comparing ourselves with others doesn't do anyone any good. And we don't really know what's going on for other people anyway. One weekend during my enforced slow down, to stave off cabin fever I took my daughter to the library. There we bumped into a newish friend of hers and her mum. We got talking about parenting and I confided that my fuse had been short lately because I hadn't been well. She told me it was understandable, but that I didn't seem like the kind of person who yelled at my kids. *You don't know the half of it*, I thought. And that's the point. So much of what we're struggling with happens behind closed doors but no one can help unless we let them in.

We know that very few women are comfortable talking to others about feeling angry in motherhood. Among the Angry Mums Club only 12 per cent spoke about it regularly with other mums. Almost a quarter had never uttered a word about frustration or fury to another mother. Indeed, there are still things I haven't felt brave enough to share in this book. But there is such a need for us to hear, as one member of the Angry Mums Club put it, stories that 'don't leave out the real

Epilogue: Am I still angry?

details of the anger'. And I see signs that this is improving. At a local shopping centre I was watching a small group of mums with toddlers having coffee near a children's play area. One cheeky kid kept grabbing sugar packets from the café table and running into nearby stores. 'Oh shit,' I heard the kid's mum say as she lurched after the toddler. She returned, out of breath, with the child in a football hold under one arm, a look of fury set on her face. Clearly at her wits' end, she deposited the kid back into the play area and picked up her presumably cold coffee. One of the other mums in the group gave her a look of solidarity and, instead of averting her gaze or changing the subject, offered a story of her own mum rage. She had recently become so frustrated during a mealtime, she confessed, that she threw something at the wall near her kid. She 'felt terrible afterwards', she told the group, and had phoned her mother for advice. (Hopefully, that grandmother offered to come around and babysit!)

This whole scene played out in a public place, mums losing their composure and sharing their frustrations unabashedly. It is also coming up more online. I've been heartened to receive emails while writing this book from mums I interviewed telling me things had improved for them. There have also been texts sharing comments from mum group chats or internet forums about angry outbursts and testing child behaviour. One in particular caught my eye, where a dad was asking for help to 'protect' his baby from a mother who yelled and screamed most days. There were the expected responses; there was 'no excuse' for that kind of behaviour and she was 'traumatising' her child. One man even said he should record his wife for evidence, leave her and take the child. But the majority of responses suggested the mum needed help. 'Could she be overwhelmed?' they asked, encouraging dad to take the baby and give her some space.

If we are going to enable mothers to speak freely about their struggles with anger, we need to make it safer to raise the red flag. We need to create an environment where the default response is support, not suspicion. Struggling mums need more avenues for help than social media and overworked GPs. The likelihood of frustration, anger and, yes, rage should be mentioned in *every* antenatal class. Every pregnant person and new parent should be screened for early warning signs. No one should be skipped over because they seem like they're coping. Lifesaving helplines and volunteer support groups need more public funding. Affordable respite through childcare should be available to all families. More dads need to start taking parental leave or asking for flexible working hours, and more employers should encourage them.

And what can we individually do? If you feel your anger is a problem, seek help. You, and your family, deserve it. Be prepared to take responsibility, learn your triggers and make changes where you can. Don't expect it to be a short, or linear, process. Be sure to repair when you can't avoid a blow-up. This is probably the most important step. In the moment, if taking a deep breath doesn't help, you could try blasting some upbeat music. I like to choose tracks with ironically relevant lyrics like Taylor Swift's 'Shake It Off' and 'You Need to Calm Down' or Meghan Trainor's 'Mother' and 'NO'. If you have little kids, you can also try focusing on their tiny hands, which has helped remind me they're not trying to break me, they're just learning.

And for others? How do we prevent another generation from only learning about all this after the fact? Nothing will change unless we are really honest. We have to warn those coming into motherhood behind us. So tell your friends, sisters, nieces, daughters, granddaughters. And, frankly, your brothers, nephews, sons and grandsons. Share your mum rage moments and take some of the shame away. If you see a mum dealing with a toddler meltdown, or swearing to herself as she wrestles a pram into the car, can you offer a hand? Could you bring snacks and a meal for the freezer to new mums instead of flowers? Could you offer time and an extra pair of hands instead of another soft toy? Because, as advocate Nadia Bergineti told me, too many of the parents who end up having their children removed by authorities could have had a different outcome if they'd had a little more of this kind of support. 'Early on, they weren't in crisis mode, they just needed a little help, and that would have changed things,' she said. 'We need to start looking at how difficult parenting is and starting from a place of parents' strengths, not just looking for the negatives. These are not parents that are trying to inflict harm on their kids. I haven't met one parent yet that has not loved their child, that has not wanted the best for them. They've just been overwhelmed.'

So, after more than a year trying to get a grip on my mum rage, do I have all the answers? Am I the poster mum for gentle parenting? Have a guess ...

I have learned a few things, though, and I hope you have too. We are not alone. We are not bad. *Some* level of anger in motherhood is to be expected. What's important is how often and why it flares, and what you do about it.

My anger is less constant, and less overwhelming these days. I still have meltdowns but I can usually pinpoint why, and reign them in more quickly. It is easier to discern when I am justifiably angry about the circumstances I find myself in (like my headache situation), and when I am being irrational or unfair (like arguments about cheese). I am better (although by no means perfect) at apologising to my kids, explaining why things got out of hand and talking about how I'd like to do better next time. (It is still a work in progress with my partner too.) There is less guilt when the rage gets the better of me, and about the tools I use to keep it at bay (like switching on *Rescue Riders*, taking antidepressants or asking for some time alone). I have been able to let go of some unhelpful expectations, which has left me with more energy to hold the line where it's really important to me.

How did I get here? Undeniably, it has a lot to do with the fact that my children are older, sleep more and are through with toilet training. It has nothing to do with any step-by-step course, journal, herbal supplement, parenting hack or gadget I ordered on the internet. Medication, reflection and communicating better with my partner have played a role. Grandparents have probably played the biggest role!

For me, it had to start with going back to basics: getting more sleep, drinking more water, moving my body and making sure I had proper meals. Only then did I have the bandwidth to reach out to professionals and make bigger changes. What have the experts and mothers in this book

Epilogue: Am I still angry?

suggested that could work for you? Could you try going to bed earlier? Tracking your cycle if you think premenstrual dysphoric disorder could be an issue? Asking your employer about flexible work arrangements? Writing your 'I Don't' list? Putting aside any spare cash to hire a cleaner? Thinking outside the box to populate your village? Giving up the gatekeeping? If you're at the end of your rope, can you just drop the rope? Don't wait too long to ask for help. Remember that good enough is enough.

And, perhaps most importantly, take a moment to give yourself a pat on the back for all the times you didn't lose your shit. Like the other night when I put my daughter to bed and, just as I crossed through her doorway, she called out 'Mum'. *Here we go*, I thought. *I've seen this episode before.* 'I'm thirsty', she said, so I circled back to hand her the cup of water on the table near her bed. As I turned to leave, I heard her shift again. Every muscle in my body tensed. *What will it be this time? She needs the toilet? She's hungry? She wants another story?* But as I glanced over, she smiled, blew me a kiss and settled down. I pulled the door closed behind me and thought how differently that could have gone. We don't acknowledge moments like that enough.

To put this book together I have sifted through reams of notes about all the times when things went pear-shaped and I wish I'd reacted differently. After a while it was starting to get me down about what a crap mum I was. So, one day, I made myself write a list of all the ways I'm a good mum. It's the sort of feel-good journalling exercise I would normally roll my eyes at, but I really needed to see the evidence in black and white. It helped. You might like to give it a go too.

My list went something like this:

I give big squeezy cuddles.
I soothe itches and ouches, tickle wriggly tummies and smooch squishy cheeks.
I gently wipe snotty noses and smelly bums.
I make endless snacks and school lunches.
I organise birthday parties and play taxi driver all over town.
I read copious bedtime stories, with all the voices.
I teach life lessons and make magic happen.
I take deep breaths. I answer, explain, listen and apologise.
I tell my kids I love them, countless times a day.

And sometimes I yell. Don't we all …

Acknowledgements

My first and greatest acknowledgement must go to the parents who shared their stories with me. This book could not exist without their honesty, courage, trust and good humour.

I relied heavily, too, on the expertise of academics, experts, frontline workers and authors (both quoted in these pages, and not) who did the work before me, opened my eyes and gave me a base on which to build.

At HarperCollins, I'm grateful to Helen Littleton for taking that first phone call before I even knew if I could (or should) do this. To Mary Rennie for taking a chance on me and understanding why this book is important. To Fiona Daniels for your thoughtful and encouraging first edit (and for stopping me from inadvertently using *that* cheese euphemism!). Madeleine James, thank you for your patience, fresh eyes, reassurance and advice on just what the manuscript needed. Thanks to Bronwyn Sweeney for your eagle-eyed proofreading, Kimberley Allsopp and Elizabeth Baral for spreading the word, Mietta Yans for a gorgeous cover design that strikes just the right vibe and Alex Wighton for keeping me in the loop. And thanks to Airlie Lawson for pushing to ensure busy, tired mums who don't have a spare hand to pick up this book could listen to an audio version.

To Lael Stone, I'm so grateful for the time you took to read my manuscript and craft such an insightful and empathetic foreword to this book – and for your encouragement during the publication process.

At *The Advertiser*, thanks to my editor Gemma Jones for allowing me the flexibility (and encouraging me) to juggle this book and my day job and never treating me differently as a part-timer. Matt Deighton, you made the connection that got this project started and have been such a generous supporter of my journalism. Each of the editors I've worked for – from the day Mel Mansell took a chance on a 17-year-old – has taught me something about good storytelling and given me the space to practice it.

I'm biased, but there's really no cooler place to work than a newsroom and no more supportive and curious crew than *The Advertiser* and *Sunday Mail* mob. Thank you to *everyone* who asked how the book was going. Cheerleaders, advisers and confidantes have included Amy Bissett, Rod Savage, Paul Ashenden, Ben Hyde, Emily Olle, Andrew Hough, Evangeline Polymeneas, Kara Jung, Brenton Edwards, Shashi Baltutis and the endlessly patient and compassionate trio of Trudie Glynn-Roe, Erin Cutler and Rachael Ormesher. (Special mentions to Jessica Leo-Kelton and Candice Keller for helping me hang in there over the years).

Writing a book is a very different game to daily news and I was grateful to be guided or encouraged by authors including Libby Trainor Parker, Ariane Beeston, Minna Dubin, Tory Shepherd, Luke Williams, Susie O'Brien, Michael McGuire and Katherine Collette. Extra thanks to Maggie Dent and Penny Moodie (for your time, and your kind words for a

Acknowledgements

debut author), Janice Orrell (for tracking down *that* book especially), Sue Shore (for lending me your office, among a few other things) and everyone in the 2026 Debut Crew.

I also needed the support of skilled professionals: Daniel Kiley, your attention to detail and willingness to talk copyright law at a brewery. Christopher Parini, your advice with numbers when I'm much more comfortable with words. Ashleigh Dumont, who captured my good side. Kate Lewis, for your clever illustration and moral support at school drop off. And feedback, fact-checking, perspective or food for thought from Yollana Shore, Toni Shore, Catherine Page Jeffery, Steve Kassem, Sylvia Gustin, Gia Hogarth, Vivienne Oakley, Dinah Thomasset and Arman Abrahimzadeh.

Immense gratitude to the patient, skilled and kind carers and educators at childcare, kindy, school and OSHC who have kept our beloved children safe and happy. It is no small act to trust strangers with the care of the most precious things in your world.

There are so many mums who have helped me through my matrescence, including AJ, Emily, Jess, Ash, Vik, Kate, Sarah, Gen, Cindy, Courtney, Julie, Jan, Leonie, Jeanine and, of course, my mum Sue. To the WAGs of the Fellowship (and your significant others), thank you for loving our two like your own. You are the embodiment of The Village. (And a shout-out to James and Paz, for enabling us moments of peace and bringing 'more energy' to your roles as honorary uncles.)

Shaun and Juliette, you enthusiastically supported this project from the start and love our kids hard.

John and Jeanine, you are always there when we need you. Thank you for all your love, support, patience and babysitting! It helps keep our family together, and I could not have written this book without it.

To my dad Greg, thank you for always encouraging me to learn and get the most out of life. (And for reading endless books to your grandchildren, who have you wrapped around their little fingers.) To my mum Sue, I don't know how many hours you've put aside to listen to my thought bubbles and grumbles. Thank you for reading everything from my school essays to the first full draft of this book (on your holiday, no less). And for warning me about the baby blues, and all the other stuff. I've wanted to be an author since I was eight years old. You and dad told me I'd need a day job, so I got one. Then, when I was ready, you helped me make this dream come true. I can't thank you enough for all you've given me.

To my partner – a private man, a patient spouse and a loving dad. I'm so grateful for our family. Thank you for sticking with me, for always being willing to try again and for unclogging the drains. Love you.

And to my sweet girl and boy, my favourite kids in the whole wide world. You were so desperately wanted, and are so completely loved. Being your mum is the *best* thing I will ever do (even if it gives me the 'irrits' sometimes). I can't wait to take you to the library to see mummy's book on the shelf.

Endnotes

Introduction
1. PwC Consulting Australia, 'The cost of perinatal depression and anxiety in Australia', November 2019.
2. Ibid.
3. Australian Institute of Health and Welfare, 'Australia's mothers and babies', 24 September 2024.
4. Consultative Council on Obstetric and Paediatric Mortality and Morbidity, 'Submission to the Royal Commission into Victoria's Mental Health System', 2019.
5. C. Thornton et al., 'Maternal deaths in NSW (2000–2006) from nonmedical causes (suicide and trauma) in the first year following birth', *Biomed Research International*, 19 August 2013, 2013(7070):623743.
6. Preventive Health SA, 'Maternal and perinatal mortality in South Australia 2022', March 2025.
7. Beyond Blue, 'New Beyond Blue data reveals people struggle for years before getting mental health support', press release, 5 October 2024.
8. Y. Stynes (host), 'Female rage – why are we so damn angry?', *Ladies, We Need To Talk*, audio podcast, 27 June 2023, ABC Listen.

It's a thing
1. Waheeda, 'Why am I an angry mom? 7 common anger triggers and how to deal with them', Messy, Yet Lovely, blog post, accessed 23 October 2024.
2. Karrie Locher (@karrie_locher), 'PP rage', Instagram, retrieved 11 November 2024.
3. A. Rich, *Of Woman Born: Motherhood as experience and institution*, Virago Press, 1976, pp.1,8.
4. S. Hays, *The Cultural Contradictions of Motherhood*, Yale University Press, 1996, p.151.
5. A. Lamott, 'Mother rage: theory and practice', Salon, 29 October 1998.

Are all the other mums yelling this much?
1. M.R. Sanders, T. Ma & E. Meester-Buma, 'National Parenting Pulse Survey: Understanding the current parenting experiences, challenges, and needs for support in Australia', *LCC Working Paper Series*, 2024-32, Institute for Social Science Research, University of Queensland, 2024.
2. Sutherbeez, 'I am filled with so much rage lately', online forum post, Reddit, 14 September 2022, www.reddit.com/r/Mommit/comments/xdz6jx/i_am_

filled_with_so_much_rage_lately/?rdt=34143; jmt20180601, 'mom rage is real', online forum post, Reddit, 12 August 2021, www.reddit.com/r/beyondthebump/comments/p2rreq/mom_rage_is_real.
3   R. Yoder, *Nightbitch*, Vintage, 2022, p.50.
4   L. Jones, *Matrescence: On the metamorphosis of pregnancy, childbirth and motherhood*, Penguin Press, 2023.
5   N. Reddy, *The Good Mother Myth: Unlearning our bad ideas about how to be a good mum*, audiobook, Pan Macmillan, 2025.
6   M. Dubin, 'The rage mothers don't talk about', *New York Times*, 13 September 2019.
7   A. Lukpat, 'These mothers were exhausted, so they met on a field to scream', *New York Times*, 23 January 2022.
8   J.E. Graham, M. Lobel & R.S. DeLuca, 'Anger after childbirth: an overlooked reaction to postpartum stressors', *Psychology of Women Quarterly*, 2002, 26(3), pp.222–33.
9   I.F. Brockington, H.M. Aucamp & C. Fraser, 'Severe disorders of the mother–infant relationship: definition and frequency', *Archives of Women's Mental Health*, 2006, 9, pp.243–51.
10 C.H.K. Ou et al., 'Seeing red: a grounded theory study of women's anger after childbirth', *Qualitative Health Research*, Oct 2022, 32(12), pp.1780–94.
11 M.R. Sanders, T. Ma & E. Meester-Buma, 'National Parenting Pulse Survey'.
12 'Child behaviour: how are Australian parents responding?', Royal Children's Hospital National Child Health Poll number 12, Royal Children's Hospital Melbourne, 17 October 2018.
13 N. Highet, 'Challenges on the journey to parenthood: what consumers had to say', Centre of Perinatal Excellence, 2019.

What is anger?
1   G. Hogarth & B. Sheridan (hosts), 'Mum rage: what it really means and how to heal – with Lael Stone', *Mum Mind Unpacked*, audio podcast, 4 June 2025.
2   D. Goleman, *Emotional Intelligence: Why it can matter more than IQ*, Bloomsbury Publishing, 1995, p.13.
3   S. Hubert & I. Aujoulat, 'Parental burnout: when exhausted mothers open up', *Frontiers in Psychology*, June 2018, 9, p.1021.
4   Y. Parfitt & S. Ayers, 'Postnatal mental health and parenting: the importance of parental anger', *Infant Mental Health Journal*, 2012, 33, pp.400–11.
5   M. Dubin, 'The rage mothers don't talk about'.
6   D. Zillmann, 'Mental control of angry aggression', in D.M. Wegner & J.W. Pennebaker (eds.), *Handbook of Mental Control*, Prentice-Hall, Inc., 1993, pp.373–74.
7   Ibid., p.379.
8   Ibid., p.380.

Endnotes

What about the dads?
1. C. Cowan et al., 'Transitions to parenthood: his, hers, and theirs', *Journal of Family Issues*, 1986, 6, pp.451–81.
2. Australian Bureau of Statistics, 'Household and families: census', 2021, released 28 June 2022.
3. J. Baxter, 'Employment patterns and trends for families with children', Australian Institute of Family Studies, May 2023.
4. J. Baxter & M. Budinski, 'Parental leave pay and dad and partner pay: patterns of use', Australian Institute of Family Studies, December 2023.
5. J. Baxter, 'An exploration of the timing and nature of parental time with 4–5 year olds using Australian children's time use data', Australian Institute of Family Studies, 2010.
6. J. Baxter, 'Fathers and work: a statistical overview', Australian Institute of Family Studies, 2018.
7. Australian Bureau of Statistics, 'Barriers and incentives to labour force participation, Australia', released 8 May 2025.
8. R. Wilkins et al., 'The Household, Income and Labour Dynamics in Australia Survey: selected findings from waves 1 to 19', Melbourne Institute: Applied Economic & Social Research, University of Melbourne, 2021.

What if you're not the 'real' mum?
1. Australian Bureau of Statistics, 'Births, Australia', 2023, released 16 October 2024.
2. N. Highet, 'Challenges on the journey to parenthood: what consumers had to say', 2019.
3. Australian Institute of Health and Welfare, 'Child protection Australia 2023–24: Supporting children: How many children were placed in unique carer households?', 25 June 2025.

It's my hormones, Doc
1. Royal Women's Hospital, 'Baby blues', retrieved 11 November 2024, www.thewomens.org.au/health-information/pregnancy-and-birth/mental-health-pregnancy/baby-blues.
2. O. Serrallach, *The Postnatal Depletion Cure: A complete guide to rebuilding your health & reclaiming your energy for mothers of newborns, toddlers and young children*, Hachette, UK, 2018, pp.42–43.
3. S. Kanowski (host), 'Jayashri Kulkarni: our hormones and our minds', *Conversations*, audio podcast, 22 February 2024, ABC.
4. J. Kulkarni, 'Premenstrual dysphoric disorder: how to treat', AusDoc.Plus, 4 September 2020.

Crying over lost sleep
1. Editors of goop, 'Postnatal depletion – even 10 years later', goop, 24 October 2022.
2. M.R. Sanders, T. Ma & E. Meester-Buma, 'National Parenting Pulse Survey'.
3. J.E. Carroll et al., 'Postpartum sleep loss and accelerated epigenetic aging', *Sleep Health*, 2021, 7(3), pp.362–67.

4   C.H.K. Ou et al., 'Correlates of Canadian mothers' anger during the postpartum period: a cross-sectional survey', *BMC Pregnancy Childbirth*, 2022, 22, p.163.
5   C.H.K. Ou et al., 'Seeing red', p.1786.
6   Ibid., p.1791.
7   Z. Krizan & G. Hisler, 'Sleepy anger: restricted sleep amplifies angry feelings', *Journal of Experimental Psychology: General*, 2019, 148(7), pp.1239–50.
8   R. Wilkins et al., 'The Household, Income and Labour Dynamics in Australia Survey: Selected findings from waves 1 to 19'.
9   S. Plage, F. Perales & J. Baxter, 'Doing gender overnight?: parenthood, gender and sleep quantity and quality in Australia', *Family Matters*, 2016, 97, pp.73–81.

Hangry mum
1   V. Swami et al., 'Hangry in the field: an experience sampling study on the impact of hunger on anger, irritability, and affect', PLoS ONE, 2022, 17(7).
2   O. Serrallach, *The Postnatal Depletion Cure*, pp.57–76.
3   'What is iron-deficiency anemia?', Johns Hopkins Medicine, accessed 23 April 2025, www.hopkinsmedicine.org/health/conditions-and-diseases/irondeficiency-anemia.
4   O. Serrallach, *The Postnatal Depletion Cure*, p.70.
5   E.R. Ellsworth-Bowers & E.J. Corwin, 'Nutrition and the psychoneuroimmunology of postpartum depression', *Nutrition Research Reviews*, 2012, 25(1), pp.180–92.

Pain in the ... everything
1   'Migraine in Australian women', Jean Hailes for Women's Health, 2025, www.jeanhailes.org.au/uploads/15_Research/NWHS25_report_migraine.pdf.
2   Australian Institute of Health and Welfare, '1 in 7 Australian women aged 44–49 have endometriosis', press release, 20 September 2023, pp.aihw.gov.au/news-media/media-releases/2023/2023-september/1-in-7-australian-women-aged-44-49-have-endometriosis.
3   B. Naylor et al., 'Reduced glutamate in the medial prefrontal cortex is associated with emotional and cognitive dysregulation in people with chronic pain', *Frontiers in Neurology*, 2019, 10, p.1110.
4   D. Kang et al., 'Disruption to normal excitatory and inhibitory function within the medial prefrontal cortex in people with chronic pain', *European Journal of Pain*, 2021, 25, pp.2242–56.
5   'Chronic pain might impact how the brain processes emotions', press release, UNSW, Sydney, 27 July 2021.
6   Y. Wang et al., 'Incidental physical pain reduces brain activities associated with affective social feedback and increases aggression', *Social Cognitive and Affective Neuroscience*, 2023, 18(1).
7   X. Li et al., 'The brain salience network at the intersection of pain and substance use disorders: insights from functional neuroimaging research', *Current Addiction Reports*, 2024, 11(5), pp.797–808.

8   N.I. Eisenberger, 'Social pain and the brain: controversies, questions, and where to go from here', *Annual Review of Psychology*, 2015, 66, pp.601–29.
9   N.I. Eisenberger et al., 'An experimental study of shared sensitivity to physical pain and social rejection', *Pain*, 2006, 126(1–3), pp.132–8.
10 Deloitte Access Economics, 'The cost of pain in Australia', 2019.

Grief and loss
1   H. Keedle et al., 'What women want if they were to have another baby: the Australian Birth Experience Study (BESt) cross-sectional national survey', *BMJ Open*, 2023, 13.
2   New South Wales Parliament Select Committee on Birth Trauma, 'Birth trauma report no. 1', 2024.
3   'Birth trauma report no.1 submission 239', Centre for Women's Health Research and Australian Longitudinal Study on Women's Health, pp.3–4.
4   'Birth trauma report no.1 submission 223', ACON, p.7; Ms Mary van Reyk, Evidence, Individual, 'Report on proceedings before Select Committee on Birth Trauma: Inquiry into birth trauma', 11 March 2024, p.6.
5   'Birth trauma report no.1 submission 932', Miss Alexandra Crichton, p.2.
6   'Birth trauma report no.1 submission 947', Aboriginal Health and Medical Research Council, p.2.
7   H. Keedle et al., 'What women want if they were to have another baby'.

We are forever changed
1   R. Wilkins et al., 'The Household, Income and Labour Dynamics in Australia Survey: Selected findings from waves 1 to 19'.
2   K. Jezer-Morton, 'Is "camel mode" inevitable for parents?', *The Cut*, 29 May 2023.
3   S. Carmona et al., 'Pregnancy and adolescence entail similar neuroanatomical adaptations: a comparative analysis of cerebral morphometric changes', *Human Brain Mapping*, 2019, 40, pp.2143–52.
4   D. Raphael, *Being Female: Reproduction, power, and change*, De Gruyter Mouton, 1975, pp.66, 70.
5   C. Conaboy, *Mother Brain: How neuroscience is rewriting the story of parenthood*, Holt, 2022, p.241.
6   E. Hoekzema et al., 'Pregnancy leads to long-lasting changes in human brain structure', *Nature Neuroscience*, 2017, 20(2), pp.287–96.
7   E.R. Orchard et al., 'Relationship between parenthood and cortical thickness in late adulthood', *PLoS ONE*, 2020, 15(7).
8   Mayo Clinic, 'Adjustment disorders', accessed 26 April 2025, www.mayoclinic.org/diseases-conditions/adjustment-disorders/diagnosis-treatment/drc-20355230.

Mothering ain't what it used to be
1   C. Pascoe Leahy, 'Maternal metamorphosis: how mothering has changed in Australia since the Second World War', *The Conversation*, 17 January 2022.
2   S. Douglas & M. Michaels, *The Mommy Myth: The idealization of motherhood and how it has undermined all women*, Free Press, 2004, p.14.

3 Ibid., p.18.
4 A. Rich, *Of Woman Born*, p.287.
5 S. Hays, *The Cultural Contradictions of Motherhood*, p.21.
6 Ibid., p.120.
7 S. Bianchi, V. Wight & S. Raley, 'Maternal employment and family caregiving: rethinking time with children in the ATUS', draft conference paper, ATUS Early Results Conference, Bethesda, MD, United States, 9 December 2005.
8 G.M. Dotti Sani & J. Treas, 'Educational gradients in parents' child-care time across countries, 1965–2012', *Journal of Marriage and Family*, 2016, 78(4), pp.1083–96.
9 N. Darnton, 'Mommy vs. mommy', *Newsweek*, 3 June 1980.
10 S. Douglas & M. Michaels, *The Mommy Myth*, p.12.
11 S.C. Flaherty & L.S. Sadler, 'A review of attachment theory in the context of adolescent parenting', *Journal of Pediatric Health Care*, 2011, 25(2), pp.114–21.
12 K. Pickert, 'The man who remade motherhood', TIME, 21 May 2012.
13 J. Winter, 'The harsh realm of "gentle parenting"', *The New Yorker*, 23 March 2022.
14 D. Serge, M. Mikolajczak & I. Roskam, 'The cult of the child: a critical examination of its consequences on parents, teachers and children', *Social Sciences*, 2022, 11, p.141.
15 S. O'Brien, *The Secret of Half-arsed Parenting*, audiobook, Murdoch Books, 2021.
16 H. Wainright, 'The "I Don't List" and why it's so important women share theirs', Mamamia, 12 August 2019.
17 C. Bowes, 'Witness History: The good enough mother', *BBC World Service*, accessed 22 June 2025, www.bbc.co.uk/programmes/w3cszmvv.
18 D.W. Winnicott, *Playing and Reality*, p.14.
19 E.Z. Tronick & J.F. Cohn, 'Infant–mother face-to-face interaction: age and gender differences in coordination and the occurrence of miscoordination', *Child Development*, 1989, 60(1), pp.85–92.

Relentless provocation
1 E. Sole, 'Mom counts how many times her kids yelled Mooooom! in a day – The total will shock you', *Today*, 24 June 2025.
2 A. House, 'Guess how many questions a mum gets asked each day', *Mamamia*, 2 April 2013.
3 G. Timothy, *Is It My ADHD?: Navigating life as a neurodivergent adult*, audiobook, Allen & Unwin, 2025.
4 ADHD Australia, 'ADHD is common, affecting one in 20 Australians', retrieved 11 November 2024; www.adhdaustralia.org.au/about-adhda.

More kids = more anger?
1 N. Reddy, *The Good Mother Myth*.
2 L. Qu, 'Families then & now: having children', Australian Institute of Family Studies, 2020.

3   J. Kingston, '"They work hard": What it's like running a household with 16 kids', Mamamia, 2 June 2019.

The self-care squeeze
1   P. Kim et al., 'Associations between stress exposure and new mothers' brain responses to infant cry sounds', *Neuroimage*, 2020.
2   A.E. Austin & M.V. Smith, 'Examining material hardship in mothers: associations of diaper need and food insufficiency with maternal depressive symptoms', *Health Equity*, 2017, 1:1, pp.127–33.
3   I. Roskam et al., 'The missing link between poverty and child maltreatment: parental burnout', *Child Abuse & Neglect*, 2022.
4   Motherly, 'State of motherhood 2024 survey report', 2024.
5   M.R. Sanders, T. Ma & E. Meester-Buma, 'National Parenting Pulse Survey'.
6   J. Couldwell & S. Pearce (hosts), 'Why being a "good enough" mother is more than enough: debunking the perfect parent myth with Dr Sophie Brock, sociologist', *Beyond the Bump*, audio podcast, 5 September 2022.

Burning out
1   S. Hubert & I. Aujoulat, 'Parental burnout: when exhausted mothers open up', *Frontiers in Psychology*, 2018, 9, p.1021.
2   I. Roskam et al., 'Parental burnout around the globe: a 42-country study', *Affective Science*, 2021, 2(1).
3   I. Roskam, M.E. Raes & M. Mikolajczak, 'Exhausted parents: development and preliminary validation of the Parental Burnout Inventory', *Frontiers in Psychology*, 2017, 8, p.163.
4   I. Roskam, M.E. Brianda & M. Mikolajczak, 'A step forward in the conceptualization and measurement of parental burnout: the Parental Burnout Assessment (PBA)', *Frontiers in Psychology*, 2018, 9, article 758.
5   Ibid.
6   M. Mikolajczak and I. Roskam, 'Am I suffering from parental burnout?', Parental Burnout, retrieved 14 September 2025, en.burnoutparental.com/suis-je-en-burnout.
7   S. Hubert & I. Aujoulat, 'Parental burnout', p.7.
8   M. Mikolajczak, J.J. Gross & I. Roskam, 'Parental burnout: what is it, and why does it matter?', *Clinical Psychological Science*, 2019, 7(6), pp.1319–29.
9   M. Mikolajczak et al., 'Consequences of parental burnout: its specific effect on child neglect and violence', Child Abuse & Neglect, 2018, 80, pp.134–145.
10 L. Hansotte et al., 'Are all burned out parents neglectful and violent? A latent profile analysis', *Journal of Child and Family Studies*, 2021, 30, pp.158–68.
11 Ibid.
12 S. Hubert & I. Aujoulat, 'Parental burnout'.
13 N. Fairbrother & S.R. Woody, 'New mothers' thoughts of harm related to the newborn', *Archives of Women's Mental Health*, 2008, 11, pp.221–9.
14 Ibid.

15 N. Fairbrother et al., 'Postpartum thoughts of infant-related harm and obsessive-compulsive disorder: relation to maternal physical aggression toward the infant', *Journal of Clinical Psychiatry*, 1 March 2022, 83(2):21m14006.
16 The Postpartum Stress Center, 'Good moms have scary thoughts', retrieved 5 December 2024, www.postpartumstress.com/speak-the-secret.
17 N. Fairbrother et al., 'Postpartum thoughts of infant-related harm and obsessive-compulsive disorder'.

Crossing lines
1 'Child Behaviour', Royal Children's Hospital National Child Health Poll, 2018.
2 Australian Child Maltreatment Study, 'The prevalence of corporal punishment in Australia', 16 June 2022, www.acms.au/the-prevalence-of-corporal-punishment-in-australia.
3 S.S. Havighurst et al., 'Corporal punishment of children in Australia: the evidence-based case for legislative reform', *Australian and New Zealand Journal of Public Health*, 2023, 47(3).
4 Y. Parfitt & S. Ayers, 'Postnatal mental health and parenting: the importance of parental anger', *Infant Mental Health Journal*, 2012, 33, pp.405, 406.

Ghosts in the nursery
1 S. Fraiberg, E. Adelson & V. Shapiro, 'Ghosts in the nursery: a psychoanalytic approach to the problems of impaired infant–mother relationships', *Journal of American Academy of Child Psychiatry*, 1975, 14(3), pp.387, 388, 420.
2 S. Kim et al., 'Mothers' unresolved trauma blunts amygdala response to infant distress', *Social Neuroscience*, 2014, 9.
3 Australian Institute for Health and Welfare, Aboriginal and Torres Strait Islander Health Performance Framework, Determinants of Health, 2.10 Community Safety, 2023.
4 Australian Institute for Health and Welfare, Aboriginal and Torres Strait Islander Health Performance Framework, Determinants of Health, 2.10 Community Safety, 2023.
5 S. Brown, 'Maternal health study: health consequences of family violence (Policy brief #2)', Murdoch Children's Research Institute, Melbourne, 2015.
6 Australian Bureau of Statistics, 'Personal safety, Australia', 2021–22, released 15 March 2023.
7 D. Haslam, 'The prevalence and impact of child maltreatment in Australia: findings from the Australian Child Maltreatment Study: brief report', *Australian Child Maltreatment Study*, Queensland University of Technology, 2023.

Being a Black mother in Australia
1 A. Lawrie, 'Holding on to our future: the final report of the inquiry into the application of the Aboriginal and Torres Strait Islander child placement

principle in the removal and placement of Aboriginal children in South Australia', May 2024.
2   Productivity Commission, 'Report on Government Services', Section F Community Services, Chapter 16 Child Protection Services, 2025.

Trying to make it work

1   J. Baxter, 'Employment patterns and trends for families with children', Australian Institute of Family Studies, 2023.
2   P. Saunders & M. Bedford, 'New estimates of the cost of children', *Family Matters*, 2018, no.100.
3   Suncorp Bank, 'Cost of kids report', 2021.
4   J. Baxter, 'Families' concerns about finances', Families in Australia Survey: Survey 3, Report no.1, Australian Institute of Family Studies, 2021.
5   Australian Bureau of Statistics, '1 in 5 Australians have experienced partner violence or abuse', media release, 22 November 2023.
6   M.R. Sanders, T. Ma & E. Meester-Buma, 'National Parenting Pulse Survey'.
7   J. Baxter, 'Employment patterns and trends for families with children'.
8   J. Baxter, 'Fathers and work: a statistical overview', Australian Institute of Family Studies, 2018.
9   Commonwealth of Australia, 'Women's Budget Statement', Budget 2025–26, 25 March 2025.
10 R. Morin, 'Study: More men on the "daddy track"', Pew Research Center, 17 September 2013, accessed 5 November 2025 at www.pewresearch.org/short-reads/2013/09/17/more-men-on-the-daddy-track.
11 J. Baxter, 'Parents working out work (Australian Family Trends No. 1)', Australian Institute of Family Studies, Melbourne, 2013.
12 M. Baird, E. Hill & S. Colussi (eds), *At a Turning Point: Work, care and family policies in Australia*, Sydney University Press, 2024, p.110.
13 'How much is a mom really worth? The amount may surprise you', Salary.com, accessed 22 June 2025, www.salary.com/articles/how-much-is-a-mom-really-worth-the-amount-may-surprise-you.
14 A. Crabb, *The Wife Drought; Why women need wives and men need lives*, Ebury Press, North Sydney, 2014, p.219–222.
15 Deloitte Access Economics, 'National working families report 2024: the impact of work and care on Australian families', 2024.
16 Motherly, 'State of motherhood 2024 survey report', 2024.
17 G. Ochiltree & E. Greenblat, 'Sick children: how working mothers cope', Australian Institute of Family Studies Early Childhood Study Paper No. 2, Melbourne, 1991.
18 J. Baxter, 'Stay-at-home dads', Australian Institute of Family Studies, 2017.
19 J. Baxter, 'An exploration of the timing and nature of parental time with 4–5 year olds using Australian children's time use data'.

The motherhood penalty

1   Workplace Gender Equality Agency, 'Gender pay gap data', retrieved 27 November 2024, www.wgea.gov.au/pay-and-gender/gender-pay-gap-data.

2   Workplace Gender Equality Agency, 'WGEA publishes new employer gender pay gaps', 4 March 2025.
3   A. Crittenden, *The Price of Motherhood: Why the most important job in the world is still the least valued*, Metropolitan Books, 2001.
4   Commonwealth of Australia, 'Women's Budget statement', Budget 2025–26, 25 March 2025, p.28.
5   H. Kleven, C. Landais & J.E. Søgaard, 'Children and gender inequality: evidence from Denmark', *American Economic Journal: Applied Economics*, 2019, vol.11(4), pp.181–209.
6   Australian Taxation Office, media release, 15 Oct 2024, www.ato.gov.au/about-ato/new-legislation/in-detail/superannuation/superannuation-on-parental-leave-pay.
7   Commonwealth of Australia, 'Women's Budget statement'.
8   Fair Work Ombudsman, 'After parental leave', www.fairwork.gov.au/leave/parental-leave/after-parental-leave.

Default parent mode
1   N. De Pisapia et al., 'Sex differences in directional brain responses to infant hunger cries', *Neuroreport*, 2012, 24.
2   J. Moser, M. Dozier & R. Simons, 'ERP correlates of attention allocation in mothers processing faces of their children', *Biological Psychology*, 2009, 81, pp.95–102.
3   J. Bick, 'Foster mother–infant bonding: associations between foster mothers' oxytocin production, electrophysiological brain activity, feelings of commitment, and caregiving quality', *Child Development*, 2013, 84(3), pp.826–40.
4   C. Scanlon, 'If fatherhood hasn't upended your lifestyle, you're not doing it right', *Sydney Morning Herald*, 25 September 2018.
5   M. Martínez-García et al., 'First-time fathers show longitudinal gray matter cortical volume reductions: evidence from two international samples', *Cerebral Cortex*, 2023, 33:7, pp.4156–63.
6   P. Kim et al., 'Neural plasticity in fathers of human infants', *Social Neuroscience*, 2014, 9(5), pp.522–35.
7   E. Abraham et al., 'Father's brain is sensitive to childcare experiences', Proceedings of the National Academy of Sciences of the United States of America, 2014, 111(27), pp.9792–7.
8   A. Rich, *Of Woman Born*, p.7.
9   S. Hays, *The Cultural Contradictions of Motherhood*, p.102.
10 N. Reddy, *The Good Mother Myth*.
11 D. Lockman, *All the Rage: Mothers, fathers, and the myth of equal partnership*, HarperCollins, 2022, p.48.
12 Ibid., p.8.
13 M. Baird, E. Hill & S. Colussi (eds), *At a Turning Point*, pp.52–56.
14 Fair Work Ombudsman, 'Minimum wages increase 3.5% from 1 July 2025', 3 June 2025, press release, www.fairwork.gov.au/about-us/workplace-laws/annual-wage-review/annual-wage-review-2024-2025.
15 M. Baird, E. Hill & S. Colussi (eds.), *At a Turning Point*, p.64.

Endnotes

16 J. Baxter & M. Budinski, 'Parental leave pay and dad and partner pay'.
17 Deloitte Access Economics, 'National working families report 2024'.
18 Workplace Gender Equality Agency, 'Parental leave', retrieved 26 April 2025, www.wgea.gov.au/parental-leave.
19 Workplace Gender Equality Agency. 'Australia's gender equality scorecard', November 2024, www.wgea.gov.au/publications/australias-gender-equality-scorecard.
20 M. Baird, E. Hill & S. Colussi (eds), *At a Turning Point*, p.58.
21 Australian Government Department of Social Services, 'Super on paid parental leave and expansion of the scheme', retrieved 12 June 2025, www.dss.gov.au/paid-parental-leave/super-paid-parental-leave-and-expansion-scheme.
22 L. Nepomnyaschy & J. Waldfogel, 'Paternity leave and fathers' involvement with their young children: evidence from the American ECLS-B', *Community, Work & Family*, 2007, 10, 4, pp.427–53.
23 M. Huerta et al., 'Fathers' leave, fathers' involvement and child development: are they related? Evidence from four OECD countries', *OECD Social, Employment and Migration Working Papers*, no.140, OECD Publishing, Paris, 2013.
24 Australian Public Service Commission, 'Maternity Leave Act review report', foreword, 2023.
25 J. Baxter, 'Stay-at-home dads'.
26 Ibid.
27 J. Baxter, 'An exploration of the timing and nature of parental time with 4–5 year olds using Australian children's time use data'.

Who said it would be 50/50?

1 *The Light We Carry*, Netflix, 2023.
2 J. Griffiths, 'A fifth of parents break-up in the year after having a baby – because of dwindling sex life, lack of communication and constant arguments', *The Sun*, 15 October 2019.
3 V. Berg et al., 'Shorter birth intervals between siblings are associated with increased risk of parental divorce', *PLoS ONE*, 2020, 15(1): e0228237.
4 R. Wilkins et al., 'The Household, Income and Labour Dynamics in Australia Survey: selected findings from waves 1 to 19'.
5 Ibid., p.97.
6 J. Baxter, 'Fathers and work'.
7 A. Woo-Ming Park, 'How some partners try to weaponize incompetence', *Psychology Today*, 30 January 2023.
8 C.H.K. Ou et al., 'Correlates of Canadian mothers' anger during the postpartum period'.
9 C.H.K. Ou, 'Seeing red', p.1797.

Dude, where's my village?

1 J. Baxter, 'Becoming a new parent in the COVID19 pandemic', Families in Australia Survey: Towards COVID Normal Report no.7, Australian Institute of Family Studies, 2022.

2   J. Baxter, 'Grandparents and child care in Australia', Families in Australia Survey: Survey 3, Report no. 3. Australian Institute of Family Studies, 2022.
3   Ibid.
4   J. Cross, 'Revealed: SA's most affordable suburbs for childcare', *The Advertiser*, 7 May 2024.
5   A. Beaini, 'Households in 20 SA suburbs fork out more than 30 per cent of median income on childcare', *The Advertiser*, 20 June 2025.
6   Productivity Commission, 'A path to universal early childhood education and care', 2024.
7   Australian Government Department of Education, 'Childcare subsidy data report – March quarter 2025', retrieved 15 September 2025.
8   Productivity Commission, 'A path to universal early childhood education and care'.
9   M. Truu, 'Labor pitches $1bn fund for new childcare centres, minimum three days subsidised care', ABC, 10 December 2024.
10 Australian Government Department of Education, 'Australian Early Development Census', retrieved 22 June 2025.
11 Productivity Commission, 'A path to universal early childhood education and care'.
12 Ibid.
13 Ibid.
14 Ibid., p.44.